Practising Quality Assurance in Social Care

Post-qualifying Social Work Practice – titles in the series

To order, please contact our distributor: BEBC Distribution, Albion Close, Parkstone, Poole, BH12 3LL. Telephone: 0845 230 9000, email: **learningmatters@bebc.co.uk**. You can also find more information on each of these titles and our other learning resources at **www.learningmatters.co.uk**.

Practising Quality Assurance in Social Care WITHDRAWN

TRISH HAFFORD-LETCHFIELD

Series Editor: Keith Brown

LEARNING
RESOURCES
CENTRE

HAVERING
COLLEGE

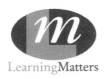

LearningMatters

First published in 2007 by Learning Matters Ltd

British Library Cataloguing in Publication Data
A CIP record for this book is available from the British Library.

ISBN: 978 1 84445 084 8

Cover design by Code 5 Design Associates Ltd
Project management by Deer Park Productions, Tavistock
Typeset by PDQ Typesetting Ltd
Printed and bound in Great Britain by Bell & Bain Ltd, Glasgow

Learning Matters Ltd
33 Southernhay East
Exeter EX1 1NX
Tel: 01392 215560
info@learningmatters.co.uk
www.learningmatters.co.uk

Acknowledgements

This book is dedicated to Alison Clark and Annie Henderson who will always be fondly remembered and their lives celebrated in awe.

Contents

Introduction

This book is about 'quality', a term that has entered the terminology of social work and social care only relatively recently, during the last two decades of the twentieth century, but which already has common currency in everyday practice. 'Quality' as a concept is multifaceted and problematic and requires a great deal of exploration and debate in order to negotiate an agreed definition of what we mean by it in the context of social care and social work services, as well as to develop the appropriate tools to measure the quality of outcomes in social care.

The successful achievement of quality within any organisation delivering social care services depends on fostering an internal culture of creativity and innovation, which takes account of its moral and ethical norms as well as the external and internal regulatory requirements. This is a complex process and the question of what works or counts as best practice in social work will probably be decided by a combination of political, social, economic and environmental influences as well as professional ones, and not least to include those identified and valued by service users themselves.

To some extent, the answers to questions about what constitutes quality in social care are already embedded in long-established and existing quality assurance systems and performance management frameworks, many of which are derived, or directly imported from, the business sector. In whichever way we encounter quality assurance and performance management systems, a practical knowledge as well as an understanding and ability to apply these concepts are inescapable requirements of all managers and practitioners in social work and social care. This can set up multiple tensions for managers who are asked to apply a straightforward business model, and such tasks can become even more complex within the current service delivery context where social care is being delivered within organisations alongside health and education and other professionals. These contexts contain a multiplicity of regulatory and performance management frameworks which can be mind-boggling to say the least.

This book aims to unpick and demystify some of the basic principles and methods underpinning the concept of quality, quality assurance and performance management systems in an interactive and developmental style. In the public sector, government plays a significant role in establishing and monitoring the standards of care against which our subsequent efforts and contributions are measured. This book seeks to redress some of this balance by inviting readers to recognise and act on those areas for which they may identify themselves as having more influence or control. This book also intends to refocus your attention to ensure that any social care service delivery and support provided remain focused on measurable outcomes for service users and carers and are driven by service user participation strategies in partnership with them.

This book was written primarily for professionals following the Post Qualifying (PQ) framework for social workers at higher specialist levels. It will be of interest to anyone following management and leadership programmes or to other professionals or practitioners working within contexts where social care is delivered and who are interested in, or have responsibility for, quality assurance in their everyday practice. Each chapter will refer to the relevant post-qualifying (PQ) standards (General Social Care Council, 2005) and the relevant Leadership and Management standards (Skills for Care, 2004a; 2006) to help you in your training and continuous professional development.

The PQ awards at higher specialist levels of social work are associated with complex decision making and high levels of professional responsibility. Higher specialist programmes are for those who have already demonstrated in-depth competence against the key roles of social work. The criteria for higher specialist social work are to:

i. Meet the academic standards for work at level M in the QAA framework.

ii. Use independent critical judgement to systematically develop their own practice and that of others in the context of the GSCC codes of practice, national and international codes of professional ethics and the principles of diversity, equality and social inclusion in a wide range of situations including those associated with inter-agency and inter-professional work.

iii. Demonstrate a substantially enhanced level of competence in a defined area of professional practice, professional management, professional education or applied professional research to the agreed national standards for higher specialist work in this area.

iv. Demonstrate a fully-developed capacity to use reflection and critical analysis to continuously develop and improve own performance and the performance of professional and inter-professional groups, teams and networks; analysing, evaluating and applying relevant up-to-date research evidence including service user research.

v. Use a critical knowledge and understanding of service user and carers' issues to develop and implement service user and carer rights and participation in line with the goals of choice, independence and empowerment.

vi. Work effectively as a practitioner, researcher, educator or manager in a context of risk, uncertainty, conflict and contradiction where there are complex challenges and a need to make informed and balanced judgements.

The management and leadership standards for social care have been developed to underpin the Skills for Care Leadership and Management strategy and can be used as a basis for developing person management specifications and to decide which learning opportunities or qualifications are appropriate for leaders and managers. The standards have been categorised using functional areas as follows:

- Functional area A: managing self and personal skills.

- Functional area B: providing direction.

- Functional area C: facilitating change.

- Functional area D: working with people.

- Functional area E: using resources.

- Functional area F: achieving results.

The topic of quality assurance and performance management thus touches on many of the standards within these areas.

Chapter synopsis

This book begins by presenting the theory base and reviews the literature and research relating to quality assurance and performance management frameworks specifically related or transferable to social care. It then goes on to focus more on the practice issues and to facilitate the practical application of concepts about quality to practice environments. We will be covering common issues and dilemmas that may arise for managers and practitioners in an organisational setting. Specific topics will be explored in line with the roles and responsibilities that you might hold in this area.

Chapter 1 gives an historical overview of the development of quality assurance and performance management in social care, charting the chronological development of national and organisational frameworks for measuring and assessing the quality and effectiveness of social work and social care services. Drawing on the policy and legislative context, there will be an examination of current inspection and regulatory regimes and a critical analysis of how far these have been effective or not. The chapter will conclude with a discussion on the future of quality assurance, inspection and regulation in social care in the context of current structural and organisational arrangements to deliver social care services in the future where these are integrated with other regulatory bodies.

Chapter 2 will further explore the different approaches to quality assurance currently adopted and recommended within the context of the public sector's managerial and political agenda. In discussing these issues, the burgeoning technical vocabulary of quality assurance, quality control and theoretical models such as Total Quality Management (TQM) will be tackled and explained. This chapter will help you to develop a more critical understanding of the value of indicators of 'quality' currently used and discuss some of the beneficial and perverse effects of trying to develop and measure these. How social care organisations go about evaluating quality at different levels and the role of managers in the various stages of the quality assurance cycle or quality chain will be discussed drawing on a range of theoretical models. The central importance of service user involvement and service user perspectives on the debate about what constitutes quality will also be covered.

As quality is an issue of organisational culture, Chapter 3 will draw on theories of organisational and workplace culture to establish the role of managers and leaders in developing team approaches to quality services. We will be looking at less tangible aspects of organisations that are considered crucial to achieving quality, for example within the concept of organisational culture. We will then go on to examine leadership theory, the differences between leadership and management, and the role of leadership in promoting quality care. Towards the end of this chapter, you will be encouraged to develop an agenda for local action by identifying areas in your particular service where there is a need for quality improvement and how you might engage your team members in this process. We will expand on such concepts as team working, partnership, motivation and delegation.

Chapter 4 will focus specifically on the role of service users in enhancing quality and continuous improvement by thinking through the different ways that we can meaningfully involve them. The needs and expectations of people who use social care services should drive changes in the way services are commissioned and delivered (CSCI, 2006) making it a priority to find out what people want and need and to involve them in how services can be developed based on their lived experiences, rather than on organisational systems and processes as illustrated above. Particular care needs to be taken to reach people who have complex needs and/or difficulty in expressing their needs. This chapter aims to look at some of the practical ways in which service user involvement, participation and control of social care services can enhance quality and continuous improvement. Starting by identifying the key principles of service user involvement, we will define terms such as 'participation' and 'outcomes' and look at the evidence for improving social care service through participation strategies. We will then identify any barriers to successfully achieving this. We will conclude this chapter by identifying methods by which managers of local services can improve accountability, transparency and openness in order to have an impact on service quality, practice and outcomes.

Chapter 5 begins by looking at the development of the evidence-based practice debate in social work and how this has been defined and characterised. We will review the limitations of evidence-based practice and the problems these raise as set out by some commentators who have questioned the usefulness and application of evidence-based practice. We will interrogate how practitioners and managers use knowledge and acknowledge the different types of knowledge-making process inherent in practice. Commitments to certain forms of knowledge can bring with them epistemological assumptions or constraints on the range of action and interventions subsequently chosen. These are important issues in the context of evidence-based practice and management in social care, given that many management techniques selected for enhancing effectiveness, efficiency and productivity reflect a set of beliefs or doctrines about how evidence-based practice should be taken forward. Chapter 6 is particularly concerned with highlighting the importance of practice wisdom and the lived experiences of service users/carers in judging the accuracy and quality of different types of knowledge and evaluation in social care following on from Chapter 5. We will conclude with some practical pointers for how you might go about undertaking your own evaluation or in-house research studies which build on knowledge and the evidence required for quality improvement and judging performance.

Chapter 6 will develop the idea that quality depends on high quality staff and the structures in place that facilitate, encourage and develop the performance of others at work. This chapter will look at the strategic drivers for workforce planning and development, and address a few of the specific areas within your own teams and services where you could have a direct impact on supporting the workforce to respond appropriately to these demands. We will also look at specific issues such as supervision, promoting diversity in workforce development and the practical challenges for sup-

porting staff who may be stressed or experience difficulties with developing competence at work.

We will conclude this book by summarising some of the most important aspects of a
quality assurance and performance monitoring system with the aim of providing you
with a quick reference guide or checklist for use in your local teams and service areas.

Websites can be a good source of further information and therefore relevant URLs will
be given at the end of each chapter, as well as references to any further or guided
reading should you wish to pursue a further interest in the topic.

Chapter 1

The development of quality assurance and performance management in social care – setting the context

ACHIEVING POST-QUALIFYING SOCIAL WORK AWARDS

If you are a registered social worker, this chapter will assist you to evidence post-registration training and learning. It relates to the national post-qualifying framework for social work education and training, in particular the national criteria at the higher specialist/advanced level.

- *ix Develop and implement effective ways of working in networks across organisational, sectoral and professional boundaries, taking responsibility for identifying, analysing and resolving complex issues, problems and barriers, promoting partnership, collaboration, inter-professional teamwork, multi-agency and multi-disciplinary communication, and ensuring the delivery of integrated and person-centred services.*

It will also help you meet the leadership and management standards for social care:

- *B1 Map the environment in which your business operates – have a clear and up-to-date picture of the environment including the 'external' operating environment – for example, customers and their needs, market trends, legislation and the activities of competitors and partners.*

Introduction

This chapter will give an historical overview of the development of quality assurance and performance management in social care by charting the chronological development of national and organisational frameworks for measuring and assessing the quality and effectiveness of social work and social care services. This overview will draw on policy and legislative contexts which have contributed to setting national standards for care and describe how these have led to the design and implementation of mechanisms to regulate and inspect social care services. You will be asked to critique the effectiveness of these latter approaches to improving or 'modernising' social care services by reviewing some of the debates about how far it is possible to design measures of quality and performance which do justice to the complexity of social work and social care services.

On the surface, the central idea behind measuring quality and performance appears to be a simple one. The theory tells us that an organisation formulates its vision about what it sets out to achieve, and then through the development of certain performance indicators, decides how this might be measured. Finally, at the end of the process of delivering a service, the organisation can then evaluate whether the expected outcome was achieved by attributing some value to this. The problem here of course, is that the effects of some interventions in social care are often difficult to measure. This is because social care is achieved through partnerships and relationships and has multiple facets (de Bruijn, 2001). Furthermore, the period between an intervention and its eventual outcome or effect may be longer term and the final effect more abstract and difficult to evaluate.

You will constantly find these types of contradictions arising throughout this book and this introductory chapter aims to establish the agenda that explains why we are so concerned with quality, inspection, regulation and performance management issues in social work and social care. The overall aim of this discussion is to help you work out your own stance towards these, based on the political, socio-economic and theoretical basis for measuring performance. This chapter will conclude with a discussion on the possible future of quality assurance, inspection and regulation in the context of the current review of structural and organisational arrangements to deliver social work and social care services.

Since the proposed and actual integration of services within a 'whole-systems' approach implemented from the beginning of the twenty-first century, regulation and inspection of social care services have become more integrated with other cross-sector regulatory bodies. Adult social care has been increasingly absorbed into health through the creation of health and social care trusts, taken further in the *Health and Social Care White Paper* of 2006. Children's services have been integrated with education following *Every Child Matters* in 2003 and the Children Act 2004. All of these initiatives have a clear focus on service user-led and defined outcomes. This is the basis for an aspirational culture in which individuals want a more secure environment and greater control in which to execute their own life plans (Webb, 2006). Social work on a par with other professionals has also achieved a much greater and knowledge and evidence base which is still growing.

However, reconfigurations of social care provision and social work services may ironically lead to social work having a much weaker presence in some of these new organisational structures. The importance of building partnerships and alliances with service users to pioneer new and different approaches to providing individual and collective support for service users has therefore never been greater (Beresford and Croft, 2004). The development of new organisational structures or enclaves is also underpinned by the notion of social inclusion, which forms an overarching concept in social policies and provides the criteria by which specific social policies are judged and evaluated. Social inclusion has also become a key measure by which social work and social care services are measured (Barry and Hallett, 1998).

Controversially, however, it has been argued that social work is abandoning a holistic approach to working with people and, as we will see later, has had to realign itself with the quasi-scientific methods of evidence-based practice and the dominant politics of how care is now managed (Webb, 2006). According to Beresford and Croft (2004), there are potential contradictions between social work presenting itself as a liberatory force on the one hand and its alliance with the regulatory or controlling role on the other. The success of social work in managing this contradiction is dependent on committed and progressive relationships between service users and practitioners which in turn act as a key component for social work reform.

When we get down to examine how these ideas pan out in practice within subsequent chapters of this book, I hope that you will be able to draw on our discussion here which will demonstrate how social work has continuously re-created itself in response to its environment. As we shall see, the greater involvement of service users, sound ethical practice and the skills of social workers in collaboration with others can together provide the potential for the profession to achieve quality in social care by cutting through any constraints and organisations – political, socio-economic or otherwise.

The development of debates about the effectiveness of social work

Post Second World War to the late 1980s

As stated earlier, the process by which social care services have come to be subject to increased scrutiny can be better understood by taking a look at the historical context and broader debates about the relationship between social policy and the development of knowledge and practice in social work. Social work and social care have been affected both directly and indirectly by changes to public services coming down from central and local government (Horner, 2003) and as the social work profession has evolved, there has been increased attention paid to what social workers actually do.

The organisation of health and social care along with the development of the British Welfare state in the late 1940s meant adoption of the standardised system of welfare created around large-scale providers of care. It was the providers, rather than the consumers, who defined the acceptability of the services provided in terms of their value for money and according to Malin et al. (2002, p124) this situation was sustained by various features of the system. For example, in the National Health Service (NHS) it was the power of the medical profession and the structure of the service itself which made it difficult for the lay public to challenge what they felt were acceptable levels of health care. In the case of social care, service providers, some of which eventually became Local Authorities (LAs), did not have the status or advantages of the medical profession. The low social status of many of their clients, and the stigma associated with receiving social care, had a similarly disempowering effect on them as consumers who were expected to be 'grateful' or 'satisfied' with the services they relied on.

In addition to this, trying to define, agree and understand what the essence or 'output' of social work was during this era was problematic. According to Clarke (1993) the origins of social care lie in its moral enterprise to control and contain certain marginal elements in society. It was only with the development of the social sciences during the twentieth century that a consideration of what outcomes one could expect from social work occurred. The emergence of modern social work was associated with the response to a number of interrelated anxieties about both the private sphere of the home and the public sphere of the state and society (Donzelot, 1988). Social work was seen by the liberal state as a positive solution to major social problems and represented a compromise between private philanthropy and the socialist vision of the all-pervasive state that would take responsibility for everyone's need. The role of the state was ultimately residual, with responsibility returned to the individual as soon as possible and the basis of any intervention was restricted to moral justification using moral guidance (Gregory and Holloway, 2005). Donzelot (1988) refers to both *moralisation*, by which he means the use of financial and material assistance to help families overcome their failures, and *normalisation*, where the provision of education, legislation and health care were tools to bring about desired changes in their behaviour and lifestyle. Social work, he said, fulfilled a mediating role between the state, mainstream society and people who were potentially excluded or disadvantaged, by taking on a gradually increasing care and control function. This grew with subsequent social care legislation and eventually became absorbed into the development of local authority social services departments in the early 1970s.

Universal state-sponsored social work and scientific approaches

The development of such therapies as psychodynamic theory and psychiatry during the 1950s onwards provided clinical modes of practice with a more scientific basis. Therapies in certain areas of social care were developed, tested and measured, and were also subject to discussion and scrutiny. Social work has always straddled these tensions; between the scientific and more humanist, client-centred approaches to practice. According to Parton (2000) although the emergence of modern social work occurred in the nineteenth century at a similar time to many of the mainstream social sciences (such as sociology, psychology and criminology and so on), even to this day, social work is seen as *newer, younger* and *less developed* (p450). The development of human sciences was concerned with looking at the nature of human beings, the reasons for their behaviour and *identifying ways in which they could be classified, selected and controlled by using scientific knowledge and professional interventions* (Parton, 2000, p457). Taxonomy approaches to concepts such as quality of life also defined key characteristics, such as those essential to good residential care. There was a number of issues identified in relation to concepts such as institutionalisation and the environmental contexts for care (Goldberg and Connolly, 1982), with a substantial critique coming from within the disability service users' movement (Oliver, 1996). In summary, during the post-war period, within the context of a new institutional framework, there was a relatively positive and optimistic view within social work about those it was working with and about what could be achieved through the casework relationship (Biestek, 1961; Stevenson, 1998).

Organisationally, legislation brought about as a result of the *Seebohm Report* in 1972 put in place large-scale and fundamental changes in structures for services in LAs. Generic social workers worked in 'patches' with maximum autonomy and responsibility for all the work in a small geographical area (Stevenson, 2005). Essential to this was a vision of neighbourhood and social networking which paid less attention to the element of social control in the social worker's role or to any need for coherent and consistent policies across particular services within local government. The limits of social work were not clearly delineated and there were many aspects of the workforce, such as home care and residential care, which had no real identification with social work. According to Stevenson (2005) the present term 'social care' to describe the workforce inclusive of social work is one outcome of this tension. It is interesting that during this period there were few standardised forms or procedures for monitoring or prescribing what social workers did, apart from the statutory documentation associated with preparing reports for courts or Boarding Out regulations for children in care (Parsloe and Stevenson, 1978). Instead, social workers operated a high degree of discretion, keeping written records only to facilitate the supervision of professional practice, as opposed to keeping an account for the outside world about what strategies they used and the subsequent outcomes or successes of these.

Radical social work

The 1960s and 1970s gave rise to criticisms of casework dominance from two principle positions. The political critique objected to the implied individualism of the method and its overall effect of taking the task of personal adjustment as the point of least resistance in the face of prevailing structural poverty and exclusion (Lyons and Lawrence, 2006). This prompted the establishment of radical social work and the rediscovery of community work which drew on the simultaneous growth of literature analysing social work and its relation to society from Marxist and feminist perspectives (Wilson, 1975; Corrigan and Leonard, 1978). Secondly, the cultural critique targeted the colour-blindness of the casework approach and its incapacity to articulate identities in collective and solidarity-constituting ways. This led to more collective approaches which analysed social problems, again using social work itself as a catalyst and reforming agent in society (Lorenz, 2006).

Simultaneously, this was a pivotal period during which interest began to focus on the actual effectiveness of social work practice. Associated with debates about predicting and assessing risk and child protection failures during the 1970s, 1980s and beyond, there were large-scale public enquiries scrutinising the effectiveness of social work (Beck 1992). These focused on its role in protecting or providing safeguards to protect children and vulnerable adults from neglect and abuse. Some commentators have noted that moral panics began from 1973, starting with the public enquiry on the death of Maria Colwell (Parton, 1985). The subsequent report (HMSO, 1974) marked the beginning of a new phase in the relationship between the public and social work, with the media as a critical intervening force (Parton, 2000).

Since then a stream of case reviews has revealed deficits and weaknesses in social work, in relation to both assessment and intervention, and the fallout of these reviews has contributed to a fall in morale in the social work workforce. It was not until the *Laming Report* (2003) that the overall stresses in which social work operates, or the quality of the management of their agencies, were sufficiently analysed. Even then, this report failed to engage with the practice dynamics that would enable a policy analysis grounded in a recognition of the emotional needs of practitioners and their organisations (Cooper, 2005).

In summary, considerable difficulties became apparent in trying to monitor the effectiveness of social work practice. Questions were raised about a lack of consensus and the ability to establish probability, cause and effect in social work intervention. Social services departments in particular were seen as unreliable institutions, with no mechanisms in place for ensuring control and the accountability of professional practitioners (Foster and Wilding, 2000).

Financial pressures also changed the climate of opinion. The economic crisis of the 1970s triggered questions about the sustainability of the Welfare State (Munroe, 2004). Slow economic growth, increased difficulties in controlling inflation, a gradual increase in unemployment, growth in the public sector and the perceived failure of social sciences to resolve social problems all provided a fertile ground for policies which brought fundamental and dramatic changes to the way in which public services were to be provided. The political environment of neo-liberalism encouraged the development of alternative approaches with a stronger theoretical basis, with a need to diagnose and solve social problems (Walker, 2002; Munroe, 2004). Underpinning this was the argument that taxpayers had the right to know that their money was being spent economically, efficiently and effectively and that citizens as consumers were entitled to monitor and demand certain minimum standards (Munroe, 2004). The government began to be explicitly interested in 'value for money' and increased the use of policies and procedures as a mechanism for prescribing how social workers should work with their clients.

This was not just the opinion of government and the public, as evaluative research and the adoption of social work professional values began to inform the training and education of social workers in the 1980s. As seen earlier, social work has always sought to maintain a critical distance from the Welfare State, despite its implicit mandate to contribute to the social, political and economic integration of those it worked with. The idea that social care could formulate clear goals and evaluate itself against these was further boosted by explicit debates on anti-discriminatory practice (Dominelli, 1988, 1989, 2002; Thompson, 2003) and the increasing influence of the service user movement (Beresford and Croft, 1980). Although this was essentially driven by moral and political interests, a commitment to achieving measurable practical outcomes was expressed. The earnest attention given to equality issues in both practice and theory in social work, and the demonstration of equality, contributed significantly to the culture of quality assurance in social care at all levels, e.g. at an individual, group and organisational level (Adams, 2002).

The development of a market economy in social care and the drive for accountability

Developments in quality assurance from 1987 to the late 1990s

The early 1990s can be viewed as a transitional period which reflected the then Conservative government's antipathy to social work and in which considerable status was given to an individualistic philosophy and to 'value for money', together with a commitment to controlling public expenditure. In many ways the early 1990s' reforms of community care policy were exemplary of the kinds of shifts in the thinking of policy-makers which introduced the market economy to health and social care via the National Health Service and Community Care Act, 1990. The White Paper which preceded the Act set out the following objectives.

- To make proper assessment of need and good case management the cornerstone of high-quality care.

- To promote the development of a flourishing independent sector alongside good-quality public services.

- To clarify the responsibilities of agencies and so make it easier to hold them to account for their performance.

- To secure better value for taxpayers' money by introducing a new funding structure for social care. (Department of Health, 1989, p5)

This provided a powerful incentive for introducing more sophisticated methods of quality and performance measurement. To meet the rising costs of care, it was felt that resources could be used more effectively by moving from a service-led to a needs-led provision (Means et al., 2003) – this move to make social services a commissioner of services and away from its traditional role as a provider had two consequences.

- That the quality and cost of care now being purchased from other agencies had to be demonstrated.

- That separate or arm's length inspection units were to be established by LAs whose specific role it was to scrutinise social services.

Both developments strongly underpin today's current focus on quality in social care, giving birth to those institutions whose role is to audit and inspect services on behalf of the government. By 2001, for example, the independent sector provided 90 per cent of residential care homes for older people and 94 per cent of homes for adults with learning disabilities (Department of Health, 2001a). A state withdrawal from direct care home provision was accompanied by strengthened state regulation of the industry. LAs and health authorities' regulation and inspection units were replaced by the National Care Standards Commission in 2002, following the introduction of the Care Standards Act in 2000. This introduced a national system of regulation based on national minimum standards with legal sanctions for those who failed to meet specified standards (Wright, 2005).

New public management and the rise of managerialism in social care

The then Conservative government was highly critical of public bureaucracies, arguing that they were dominated by self-serving interests and were unresponsive to users' needs (Henkel, 1991, p11, cited by Munroe, 2004). This led to a set of measures aimed at bringing professionals under tighter managerial control, with more emphasis on professional management, the introduction of explicit measures of performance, a focus on outputs and results and an ever greater role played by private sector styles of management practice. Pollitt (2003) draws specific attention to the changes that took place which involved privatisation, contracting out and bringing the internal market or 'quasi-market' into the social services and the NHS. The outcome of these reforms has been the creation of a new set of principles which govern practices in the public sector, which Ferlie and Steane suggest all boils down to *managers, markets and measures* (2002, p1461).

Managerialism and the language of consumerism

Gregory and Holloway (2005) capture the changes brought about in this era through their analysis of a common language which has since been adopted by the social work profession. Community care has become an 'enterprise' shot through with consumerist and market-management terminology and the very term for the vehicle prescribed to deliver this new community care – 'care management' – both reflects the managerial culture and is linked irrevocably with the ideologically-driven changes in the arrangements and underpinning principles for health and social care. The implication of this language is that care is a 'commodity' to be managed like any other, and the recipients of care are 'consumers' of the product. The theorising of the models of care management and the analytic frameworks used for service evaluation hammer home the message. For example, Challis et al. (1998) borrow from economics the term 'vertical integration' (structures to describe the health and social care interface) and the care manager becomes a 'social entrepreneur' who stimulates resource provision so as to make possible a flexible creative response to individual need. This managerial, outcome-focused influence is particularly evident in the discourse about quality. According to Gregory and Holloway, it is no accident that the emergence of 'quality talk' has been simultaneous with the community-care changes. As with the drive for reform in community care, its roots were in an increasing transposition of a business ethic and business practices into the human services in the 1980s with the language of commerce giving rise to language of quality assurance in social-care agencies. (Gregory and Holloway (2005, p48–9)

A centralisation of power and decision-making by successive governments in the late 1990s had major consequences for the way in which practice is now managed. Not only are social care organisations expected by government to manage services efficiently and effectively, they must simultaneously manage the quality and effectiveness of direct work with service users and carers. This has caused tensions and dilemmas for both managers and practitioners. The redesign of organisational frameworks took place to give clarity and increase the effectiveness of the way in which services are assessed and provided for. These have also subtly taken over the exercise of professional skill and decision-making as increasing expectations of service users conflicting with the demands and constraints of the social care system meant that large bureaucracies, for example in statutory settings, could no longer respond flexibly (Kearney, 2004, p104).

ACTIVITY 1.1

What examples can you think of where social work decisions are strongly influenced by the existence of policies and procedures? What areas of your current work are subject to regulation and inspection and what effect, if any, does this have on your service's relationship with users/carers?

Beresford and Croft (2004) have identified four key influences on social work during this period which characterise this increasing trend of social work's role as a means of state control.

- Social work's loss of identity.
- The devaluing of social work practice.
- The dominance of ideology and managerialism.
- Globalisation and social exclusion. (Beresford and Croft, 2004, p56)

The examples you come up with may fall under the above influences. One example might be where you supervised staff in undertaking a complex process to assess a person's need for support and care and then did not have the authority to sanction the resources or process to take this forward. Perhaps there was a separate resource panel for decision-making which subsequently prioritised different interests over those that your team sought to promote for the service user.

The development of regulation and performance measurement from 1997 to the twenty-first century and the development of outcome-based cultures

As discussed earlier, the partial withdrawal of the state from direct provision of welfare services and the giving of more responsibility to the independent sector to provide care on their behalf have given rise to a substantial growth in the regulation and control of all services. We will see later this has had particular consequences for the previously more independent role of the voluntary sector and on their ability to enter the market in the first place. Implications have been far-reaching. Regulation through contracting, monitoring and inspection is symptomatic of wider cultural changes and the development of what is referred to as an *audit* society (Means et al., 2003).

CASE STUDY

In 2004, an inquiry by the King's Fund examined the way in which care services were provided for older people in London. They identified that effective local partnerships between the public and independent sectors can offer support to small voluntary organisations willing to develop home care services for particular minority ethnic groups. However, practical support for small voluntary organisations was, in some cases short lived, as the authorities concerned changed their policies and bought 'more of the same' kinds of community services operating within separate silos.

Recommendations were made to use public money innovatively, such as by providing a care business development service, supported by health and social care organisations. This could support the building of new business in local communities to drive innovation and stimulate a more flexible and versatile range of home care services which would deliver better integrated services for older people. (Robinson and Banks, 2005, p120–1)

The incoming Labour government of 1997 brought with it a complex and interlocking set of reforms intended to transform the regulatory framework for social care and improve performance in every area. These initiatives formed part of new Labour's agenda for local government in 'modernising' public services and represented a significant increase in the involvement of central government in the direct management and delivery of services. The *modernising social services* framework (DoH, 1998) stressed the importance of raising service quality and consistency, highlighting the differences between the objectives of social care and the actual standards achieved. Both these and other concerns about the performance of social services have led central government to adopt an increasingly interventionist stance towards regulation of the sector. This change was most marked with the introduction of new legislation such as the Care Standards Act 2000 and Community Care (Delayed Discharges) Act 2003 together with a greater thrust towards increasing central government regulation over both policy content and the policy process (Means et al., 2003). By defining the core business of social care through more systematic procedures and coercive management techniques, it has been speculated that the process of dialogue between the state and the social work profession has continued to change dramatically (Jordan and Jordan, 2000; Jones, 2001).

A quality strategy for social care

According to government guidelines, the quality of social care services is a local responsibility which can be delivered only if there is radical change at a local level. This will be achieved by a number of means.

- Implementing Best Value, which will drive continuous improvement in the way services are provided by local authorities.

- The introduction of a framework to ensure continuous quality improvement, which emphasises the importance of staff development and training together with high standards of practice at all levels.

- Actively fostering a culture within social services that emphasises lifelong learning.

- Creating a sound evidence-base from which to drive service change.

- Generating and cementing creative partnerships between all sectors and across all fields, to develop innovative and flexible services.

- The imaginative use of information technology.

- Regular and rigorous assessment of local councils' performance in achieving these goals. (DoH, 2000a, p21)

ACTIVITY 1.2

So far we have been looking at the historical context where I have presented a perspective which deliberately highlights a strong managerialist stance towards improving services. Of course, this is not the only perspective and I would like you to think about other viewpoints that have also emerged over the last decade from service users/carers and professional social work practitioners.

ACTIVITY 1.2 *continued*

What other triggers can you think of that have been active in driving the improvement of services? Can you give any examples of research or evidence in your area of practice for which you have responsibility which have informed policies towards improving outcomes for people using or on the receiving end of services?

The table below shows some of the key policy initiatives which have reinforced quality assurance approaches and performance management in social care. You may have already identified the role of registration and the training of social workers, plus the links between learning from research and the greater involvement of the service user movement in education, training and the direct delivery of services.

Table 1.1 Key policy initiatives related to quality in social care

Initiative	Lead Agency	Objective
Best Value (1999)	Local government	Method of systematically reviewing and evaluating Services based on the 4 'Cs': *Challenge* – why the service is needed *Compare* – cost and quality with 'like' services *Consult* – with public and service users to test the validity of conclusions *Compete* – to ensure the best way of providing
Quality Protects (1999)	LAs	Improve and develop services provided to vulnerable children defined by the Children Act 1989. Outlines 11 objectives for children's services. Has performance criteria and indicators against which LAs assess themselves towards MAPS (Management Action Plans).
National Service Frameworks	NHS and LAs	Brings together a coherent set of national standards aimed at providing national standards and objectives for social care in specific service user groups. These are holistic and build on collaboration between relevant agencies to provide quality services, which promote health and well-being.
National Care Standards Act 2000	CSCI	Legislation setting out national minimum standards against which providers are registered, inspected and regulated.
Quality Strategy for Social Care 2000	General Social Care Council	Statutory agency established to regulate and register the social care workforce and a national code of practice and conduct for all social care employers and employees.
	Social Care Institute for Excellence	Organisation responsible for developing and disseminating the knowledge base for social care and providing an accessible electronic database about best practice.
Fair Access to Services (2002)	NHS and LAs	Method of testing eligibility for services using four categories which help to avoid geographical variations in assessing needs and risks as *critical*, *substantial*, *moderate* and *low*.

National service standards

You will also have noticed from Table 1.1 that there has been a specific drive to set national standards for social care. The introduction of national minimum standards over the last decade has established different sets of standards for different care services including those in the statutory, private and voluntary areas of health care in England. National minimum standards involve extensive analysis of the quality of care that must be provided by specific services and define these in a way than enables them to be measured for quality or to identify shortfalls in provision.

Key characteristics of a service standard

- It can be measured, monitored and evaluated.
- It's realistic and attainable within available resources.
- It's expressed clearly and unambiguously and tells people what they can expect.
- It's consistent with service aims and values.
- It's set in conjunction with the people asked to achieve it.
- It reflects what people say they value most. (Martin and Henderson, 2001, pp194–5)

Later on in this book we will identify what might constitute appropriate measures for the effectiveness of social work and will utilise some of the national service standards from different service user groups to test out techniques for objectivity and subjectivity using qualititative and quantitative measures. In the meantime we will concern ourselves mainly with the way in which national service standards are used to measure outcomes within the current performance management regime. Hopefully you will agree that service standards and minimum care standards incorporate many of the aspirations and individual values of social work and should therefore be owned by those delivering services against these as an essential part of their practice values rather than just as tools for external inspection. National standards are seen by government as an important tool by which to measure and chart progress, particularly within statutory organisations, and we shall now look at some of the ways in which this takes place.

Inspection regimes and performance assessment frameworks

Star ratings for social services were announced in 2001 as a means of summarising an inspection body such as the Commission for Social Care Inspection (CSCI) or the Audit Commission's independent judgement of performance across all social services on a scale of zero to three stars. This is part of the current Labour government's comprehensive Performance Assessment Framework (PAF), where the allocation of ratings aims to improve public information about current performance of services and their capacity for improvement at local, regional and national levels.

These ratings are supposed to provide an objective starting point for reviewing and planning improvements to services and are contingent on good social services' inspections. Authorities performing well have more freedom in the way they use their centrally-provided grant funds with reduced programmes of inspection and monitoring. Authorities with zero stars are subject to more frequent monitoring and have special monitoring arrangements and additional support put in place. Examples of Personal Social Services (PSS) and PAF indicators you might come across in your local councils are:

- indicators to demonstrate that people from minority ethnic groups are treated fairly;
- providing services at a reasonable cost;
- investing now to prevent people needing more services later;
- helping to promote older people's independence.

Star ratings are designed to be compatible with the performance information and ratings of the NHS and other local government services. They are based on an amalgamation of all PIs in that authority. A PI is one of the ways in which the government measures how a national standard has been achieved. Many PIs are targeted at measuring how social care is integrated with other services.

Integration of social care – a good practice example

Strong relationships between North Tyneside Youth Offending Team and social services were reported during inspections. This includes a protocol with social services in relation to looked-after children, court work and remands to council accommodation. In the cases sampled, social services were always involved during the supervision period for looked-after children and those considered vulnerable from self-harm. Difficulties in relation to the placement of children and young people in local accommodation were being actively addressed. There were also effective arrangements for information-sharing between the Courts and the Youth Offending Team: Youth Offending Team Court Officers have access to an office and a networked terminal in the Courts so that Court Orders can be processed quickly. (CSCI, 2005a, p80)

The PAF requires social services authorities to translate their labours into numbers, such as the unit cost for each resource, the percentage of looked-after children who are adopted, and the number of elderly and disabled people helped to stay in their own homes (DoH, 1999b). This means that an examination of social workers' individual caseloads is not enough to make quantitative judgements about whether particular LAs are getting enough children in or out of care or the child protection system. These have to be benchmarked against what others have achieved in similar circumstances and within the standards expected.

ACTIVITY 1.3

What difficulties, if any, can you identify with this approach? What other factors are present when measuring or assessing the success or achievement in meeting a quality standard? You may wish to take one from your own service area to help you in this exercise.

You may have identified that there are many contradictions in this approach. First of all, not all service user groups are covered by legislation and policies that exist to set standards and improve services. Children in the asylum process constitute one such group where there are anomalies between the new legislation aimed at improving the welfare and safety of children under Clause 11 of the Children Act 2004 and the tighter controls on immigration which may have harmful effects on children (Humphries, 2004; Hudson, 2005). Young people in the youth justice system are another example, as research has shown that those in young offenders institutions are at the greatest risk of bullying, intimidation and self-harming behaviour, yet fall outside the scope of the new legislation (Hudson, 2005). Other contradictions in this approach will be explored in Chapter 2 when we unpick some of the models and terminology involved in measuring quality and thus performance.

Many commentators have argued in some detail that social work should take a broader view of its remit, to include economic activity, social regeneration, community work and many projects still unfamiliar to the social work profession (Jordan and Jordan, 2000; Lymbery and Butler, 2004). Clarity is also needed about social work's position in relation to the new organisational structures it will operate within. Despite these changes, many of social work's central tasks will remain familiar: the concern with rights and justice linked to the life cycle; circumstances; relationships between individuals; families and communities; health and disability. Jordan and Jordan (2000) argue that the biggest threat to optimism for the future of the social work profession lies in the specific mindset about practice which fits in with top-down policy prescription and accountability, with the ad hoc developments of solutions to particular problems, with targets and standards, and with the obsession with effectiveness and value for money that the New Labour government inherited from its predecessors (p205). Jordans' discussion of 'tough love' (meaning the capacity to communicate optimism and energy in the solution of problems, and the confidence that service users can be supported to realise their potential) describes the tensions within the very technical methods and measures for addressing particular needs and objectives, providing *a dreary, mechanistic, systematic , technocratic approach that puts clients in categories and produces a ready-made package according to a pseudo-scientific classification of their deficits* (2000, p205).

The influence of research and evidence-based practice on measuring effectiveness

As we have seen, the modernisation of social care places a high premium on evidence and, at the level of central government commitment to service reform, is increasingly based on evidence about effectiveness rather than on any partisan political agenda.

According to Marsh et al. (2005) at the level of service users or citizens, the acceptance of professional expertise should be supported by access to high-quality information. At the level of service providers, accountable and regulated services should also ensure that practice is based on evidence rather than on past practice or current patterns of practice. Despite this vision, only 0.3 per cent of the current government's annual spend in research and development is in social care (compared with 5.4 per cent in health: see Marsh et al., 2005, p.*xi*). This points to a need for a research infrastructure that is capable of supporting an evidence base of sufficient quality to underpin national policy-making and to develop practice knowledge (Marsh et al., 2005, p1).

Marsh et al. (2005) propose six main arguments for the need for evidence from research within the knowledge base for social care.

1. The major impact of the decisions of social care professionals on the immediate life chances of services users and carers (e.g. in child protection) as having the best informed practitioners is vital to the immediate outcomes for highly disadvantaged people.

2. The impact over time of decisions on the longer-term life chances of service users and carers (for example looked-after children). Best informed practice should be the right of people whose long-term outcomes and quality of life depend in part on social care decisions.

3. Good evidence may challenge fundamental assumptions about social care, and bring substantial advantages to service users and carers. Research can aid major and sometimes controversial shifts in policies, which have the potential to enhance greatly the lives of service users and carers, for example on direct payments.

4. The importance of providing safeguards over compulsory or quasi-compulsory decisions, for example where professional or legal powers are used to make decisions in major aspects of people's lives. Providing the best available evidence is an important component of these processes of social control.

5. The need for an informed public who can engage in active and relevant debates about services.

6. The need for informed service user and carer communities and individuals that promotes direct involvement in services and engagement with their development (Marsh et al., 2005, pp3–4).

We will be looking further at some of these issues later on in this book when we examine the opportunities for evaluating services and developing *communities of practice* where staff learning and development can be maximised (Wenger, 1998). The role of prevention is equally valid and was only recently made explicit in the Adults' Green Paper, *Independence, Wellbeing and Choice, 2005.* Whilst considerable resources have been made available for protection or safeguarding in social work and social care, the development of preventative services has been given little attention in terms of either research or funding (ADSS, 2005).

CASE STUDY

Prevention – providing an integrated falls service for older people

The Department of Health (2000b) define an integrated falls service as one which comprises:

1. Agreeing and implementing local priorities to reduce the incidence and risks of falls.

2. Ensuring appropriate initial assessment and response (for example to an emergency department or through intermediate care services, where the need for hospital assessment is not required) to those who have fallen.

3. Having a multi-disciplinary falls team, so that people with recurrent falls, or one fall with serious consequences, have access to specialist assessment to identify and reduce risk for further falls and manage the consequences of the fall.

4. Having an osteoporosis service, and in particular diagnostic scanning, to reduce the risk of osteoporotic fracture and long-term impact of falls.

5. Having rehabilitation services for those who have lost functional ability or confidence after a fall.

An inspection by the Healthcare Commission, CSCI and the Audit Commission in 2004 reviewed progress made by the NHS, LAs and partners in meeting the standards set out in the National Service Framework for Older People and the impact this has had on the lives of older people. Many of the inspections found a lack of investment in services to address falls, with little commitment beyond replacing ill-fitting slippers. The role of LAs in making sure that pavements and public areas are safe, providing improved lighting, fitting stair rails in a person's house and in offering opportunities for exercise to improve strength and balance was not recognised as part of a whole-system approach to the prevention of falls.

> 'Mum had one fall but I didn't know how to contact people. The second time she fell I had the control centre number and they rang my mum on the intercom. She fell again and the paramedics came. Services were going to be arranged when she was discharged, but then they decided she would go into a home' (carer's feedback).

(From a review of progress against the National Service Framework for Older People, CSCI, 2005b, p58)

Politically-inspired changes to the reorganisation of services have arisen from some of these dissatisfactions with the performance of social services departments, especially in relation to the welfare of children. Current initiatives set out in the *Health and Social Care White Paper* (2006) and *Every Child Matters* (DfES, 2003) and supported by the Children Act 2004, aim to bring social services for children together with education, health and the independent sector. The creation of 'children's centres' is part of the wider agenda to ensure that a range of agencies and workers act together more effectively to safeguard children. Stevenson (2005) argues that these contain an implicit rejection of the value of one generic social service agency base from which social workers operate, and may drive an even deeper wedge between social work services in different specialisms (e.g. mental health and child protection) which are frequently at the root of situations in which children's safety is jeopardised (p576). Furthermore, Stevenson argues, the location of preventative services such as SureStart in agencies outside departments in which child protection services are placed creates a division at the level of work with families which has major implications for continuity of care.

As we saw earlier, organisational change and restructuring over the last 20 years have been dictated by the perceived need to reorganise the work for greater efficiency, largely as a symbol of change and progress, with little long-term evaluation of the benefits or the creation of opportunities for emerging professionals to develop their identities within an increasingly controlling management agenda. Managerialist systems have not, by and large, created a climate of trust and enthusiasm or structures which encourage dynamic and imaginative practitioners (Dominelli, 2002). Without such opportunities, social work expertise cannot be developed and quality cannot be enhanced.

The future of regulation, inspection and performance measurement in social care

From our examination so far, you will appreciate that performance management and regulation are integral to our organisations and firmly enshrined in legislation and policy. The future of social care regulation set out in the *Better Regulation Task Force* (Better Regulation Commission, Cabinet Office 2004) emphasises the current government's intention to increase the participation and contribution of users in the process of inspection and regulation. Sections 20–24 of the Children Act 2004 require an integrated inspection framework to be established by the relevant inspectors to inform future inspections of all services for children. This implies a coordinated approach by a wide range of inspectorates or 'super-inspectorates'. Ofsted will be the lead inspectorate, working closely with the Commission for Social Care Inspectorate (CSCI), the Healthcare Commission and the Audit Commission. However, a further six inspectorates will likely have involvement: the Adult Learning Inspectorate; HM Inspector of Constabulary; HM Inspectorate of Probation; HM Inspectorate of Prisons; HM Magistrates' Courts Services Inspectorate and HM Crown Prosecution Service Inspectorate (Hudson, 2005). According to Hudson, not only will there be a common strategic approach, but individual inspectors will increasingly be working in multi-disciplinary teams – a formidable task to coordinate. This Joint Area Review process will *describe what it is like for children and young people growing up in the area and evaluate the way local services, taken together, contribute to their well being* (Ofsted, 2004, para 6, cited in Hudson, 2005). Hudson thus concludes;

> *Agencies invariably skew their behaviour to ensure they meet the criteria upon which they are judged, so that any deficiencies in inspection and performance managing will have a significant knock-on effect on service organization and delivery. The changes that will be brought in by the new integrated inspection framework are immense and complex and it would be surprising to find no gap between policy and implementation . . . although*

> *described as 'transformational' . . . the rational top-down approach being*
> *taken by central government displays insufficient appreciation of the*
> *importance of 'bottom-up' implementation factors.* (Hudson, 2005, p518)

For adult services the new arrangements for regulating and inspecting health and social care will need to focus equally on inclusion and participation, supported by effective transport, leisure, housing and other council-led functions and the independent sector. However these arrangements transpire, a number of new expectations will be placed on regulation and inspection regimes in that they must focus more on outcomes, which in turn means looking at how services deliver for their users. Finally, at a local level, the motivation to cooperate should be sustained by good inter-organisational and external relationships and obligations which take on board both moral and ethical values as well as regulatory ones.

C H A P T E R   S U M M A R Y

In this chapter we have been given a brief overview of how quality assurance and performance management systems have been established in social care by identifying the key initiatives and policies that successive governments have put in place as an attempt to ensure that standards of care improve and that social work practice can be scrutinised and regulated. We have touched on ideas about evidence-based practice as being fundamental to developing and achieving outcomes for service users. This has, however, created some tensions between the social work profession and their regulators about what constitutes an evidence-based approach. We will return to this debate in more detail in Chapter 5.

What is important about understanding the basis for what constitutes a quality service or good performance in social care is the emphasis on locating practice within the context of social relations and how these ideas have come about within the political and economic setting. There has been criticism of narrowly-conceived studies of quality and performance in particular settings, which see *social work activity as the delivery of a set of pre-packaged responses to need that can be broken down into minutely specified elements and then recombined in many different forms* (Jordan, 2002, p205). The danger in this approach is caused by reducing social work to a form of practice that can be implemented through a set of detailed guidelines and instructions from government advisers and researchers alone, resulting in lost opportunities for innovation or creativity in developing quality care.

As we have seen, successive governments have created huge pressure on social services organisations to deliver against centrally-defined objectives, and whilst the general antipathy of the Conservative government in the 1980s to notions of public services has been replaced by New Labour's predilection for regulation and performance, overall outcomes have been similar. Organisations in social care have had to adjust to ever-increasing levels of external scrutiny. According to Lymbery and Butler (2004) this has fostered an inherently defensive attitude within many organisations, constraining the activities of social work practitioners and aiming towards more *defensive social work practice* (Harris, 1987). Pressure on practitioners to accept rather than challenge the limitations of policy can prevent them recognising the relationship between process and outcomes in social work which legitimises good practice and rebuilds confidence within the profession. Reaffirmation of the belief in a model of social work in which interpersonal skills, grounded in theory and knowledge, presides is at the heart of providing quality services. We will be exploring these less tangible issues later in this book, after we have got to grips with the literature, concepts and common techniques used to measure quality and to develop quality assurance systems in social care – which will be the topics of our next chapter.

FURTHER READING

Jordan, B and Jordan, C (2000) *Social work and the third way: tough love as social policy.* London: Sage.
This book offers a lively debate and analysis on the relationships between New Labour's programme of reform and the implications for social work practice.

Webb, S (2006) *Social work in a risk society: social and political perspectives*. Palgrave Macmillan.
This book focuses on the evolving role of social work practice and how it relates to the ever-present phenomenon of risk. It highlights and debates current tensions and trends for social work as a consequence of increased regulation and state control and suggests ways of rethinking models that are more ethical and professional.

Commission for Social Care Inspection
The main body that regulates social care in partnership with other agencies and which will be integrated with Ofsted in 2008. CSCI publishes a number of studies on outcomes of their work in different service areas. These are available at: **www.csci.org.uk**

Department of Health
The following government publications can be obtained from the DoH website (**www.doh.gov.uk**) and will give you more information on the strategic outcomes for both adults' and children's services as well as updates and guidance on how these are being implemented and progressed.

Independence, well-being and choice: our vision for the future of social care for adults in England (2005)

Every Child Matters: change for children (2003)

Chapter 2
Quality assurance – theoretical models

Introduction

In the previous chapter we identified that enhancing quality has been increasingly emphasised as a key goal for the personal social services and their organisations in the UK over the last decade. Achieving quality in service delivery is an integral part of, and justification for, many of the initiatives emanating from the government's modernising agenda (DoH, 1998). Integrated within the approach taken by government, the key to improving quality is one where tasks in social care are more clearly defined, accompanied by an assessment process to ensure that these requirements are met in practice. Underpinning this stance is an assumption that developing quality is a technical, value-free activity which merely requires good management combined with encouragement and a commitment to implement and be effective in its application (Watson, 2004). However, as we will see, developing quality is a much more complex activity than merely defining and measuring performance and there is a clear view that performance measurement in itself does not do any justice to the nature of activities performed by public sector organisations (de Bruijn, 2001). The complexity and multiplicity of activities that contribute towards delivering social care services for example are often unpredictable.

In contrast, many approaches to performance measurement tend to reduce such complexities to a single dimension; for example, achieving set targets may not tell us anything about the professionalism and/or quality of the performance during the process of delivering a service or how it may even have been detrimental within these parameters. It is worth acknowledging here that some research studies substantiate how the vast majority of people working in social care are genuinely concerned about the quality of the service they provide (Healey, 2002; Weinberg et al., 2003; Watson, 2004), therefore striving for quality is a key motivational factor for employees and a concept that managers or people responsible for implementing quality can build on, inextricably tied up with workforce development (DfES/DoH, 2006). A well-designed quality service can empower and support employees in making service improvements, particularly when it leads to direct benefits for them, such as increased job satisfaction, reduced frustration, and being in receipt of better feedback from the people they work alongside as the reputation of their service or organisation improves.

The overall aim of this chapter is to look at the numerous concepts and theories associated with 'quality', without this becoming a mere academic exercise. To achieve this we will acknowledge how the theoretical base can help us to develop a practical approach to delivering quality services. We will begin by defining what we mean by quality and its different dimensions. Given the tendency to adopt buzzwords or jargon in the health and social care sector around quality and quality assurance, we will try to unpick these terms and clarify exactly what is meant by them. We will, for example, examine what is meant by terminology such as 'quality control', 'quality assurance', 'total quality management' and 'excellence', so that we can appreciate the differences between these terms and consider how useful or applicable they are to us in social care.

This chapter will also help you to develop a more critical understanding of the value of developing indicators of 'quality' by exploring some of those commonly used in social care and we will also discuss some of the beneficial and perverse effects of trying to measure these. The central importance of service user involvement and service user perspectives on the debate about what constitutes quality will also be mentioned, although we will be addressing these more fully in Chapter 4. This chapter will conclude with an exploration of how ideas and principles in social work and social care can become compromised or in conflict with external social, economical and political pressures on the organisational performance agenda. This will lay the ground for us to do more practical work on the role of advanced practitioners and managers in making quality assurance a reality in their specific areas of responsibility, which will then be explored in the remainder of this book.

Defining quality

Quality is an elusive concept which has a number of different meanings and variants of meaning that are difficult to entangle. In part this is due to the different settings in which the term is applied (Patel, 1994). Everybody talks about quality as if a common understanding exists but the reality is that this can vary from organisation to organisation and between different stakeholder groups. Yet achieving a common definition is important, as it drives the whole implementation process and is the basis of standards setting and measurement (Gastor, 1995d). Various dictionary definitions and those offered by quality 'gurus' are generally seen to be value-orientated; for example *delighting the customer by fully meeting their needs and expectations* (www.dti.gov.uk/quality/) or *the totality of features or characteristics of a service that bears on its ability to satisfy a given need. It must be explicitly designed and built into a service; it cannot be inspected at the time of, or after, delivery* (Davies and Hinton, 1993, p51).

These commonly accepted definitions clearly indicate that quality is ultimately judged on the customer's perception of how a service met their needs.

Before going further, you will have noticed that I have introduced the term 'customer', whereas in social care we tend to use the term 'service user' (or at the time of writing, the term 'expert by experience' has been adopted when referring to the specific involvement of service users in inspecting or advising on quality issues). Authority comes to language from outside in the social world and the particular meanings we attach to words reveal the underlying values and attitudes about the things to which we are referring (Pugh, 1996). Because social work is intrinsically tied to social and economic change, political activity can have a huge impact on the language adopted by social work and social care professionals (Heffernan, 2006). This is most certainly true in the area of quality and performance management. This chapter will refer mostly to people utilising social care support and services as 'service users'; however it has been proposed that the term 'service user' often means a 'consumer' or 'customer' of social care services which is why we sometimes see these terms used interchangeably (Heffernan, 2006). As we saw in the previous chapter, much of the language associated with quality originates within the political ideologies and the consumerist model of social care, which in turn has presented many challenges where there is a lack of resources or choice of services. It is important to acknowledge the political context for transferring these concepts and we will return to this issue shortly. First of all we are going to try and define exactly what we mean by quality.

We probably all know from first-hand experience what we consider to be either a poor-quality or a high-quality service. Moullin (2003, p13–14), however, offers us four definitions of quality derived from the management literature.

- **Fitness for purpose** – if an item or service fits the purpose for which it is intended then it is said to be a quality product.

- **Conformance to specifications** – the item or service reflects both the views of professionals and the needs and expectations of service users and is based on an accurate specification of what is required.

- **Conformance to requirements or responsiveness** – by providing exactly what the customer needs at the right time and in the right way.

- **Meeting customer requirements at an acceptable price** – this definition is based on a consumer model where the customer's concept of quality matters most and it is a question of being responsive to their full range of needs and assisting in the fulfilment of those needs.

ACTIVITY **2 . 1**

How do the above definitions accord with the circumstances of social work and social care and the expectations of its users/carers? Can you identify any issues or challenges in meeting the terms implied within these definitions by referring to practical examples of services or service activities from your own area of responsibility?

The 'products' being specifically discussed here in relation to quality are those concerned with the direct delivery of care and support services to users, carers and the community. These include social work activities in statutory organisations, where the latter are responsible for providing protection or social control with particular groups in society as a result of its legislative duties (Dalrymple and Burke, 2003). Within this context, 'quality' can be seen as a potentially ambiguous concept. Any definition adopted is subject to interpretation and trade-offs between the needs of an organisation and its 'customers' and these may be played out in situations where some stakeholders will have more power than others.

For example, in non-profit making enterprises, resource constraints and the need to prioritise particular service user needs over others both have the potential to compromise the quality of service users'/carers' experiences or the extent of the service provided. Normann (1978) defines this as the *moment of truth* (cited in Moullin, 2003). By this he means that the quality perceived is realised at the moment when the service provider and the service customer confront each other, leading to three possible outcomes: firstly, the customer will get less than they expect and be disappointed or angry; secondly, the customer will get exactly what they expect and are satisfied; and thirdly, the customer gets service of a higher quality than they expect and is therefore delighted. You will no doubt find this scenario familiar in day-to-day encounters with service users and particularly in the decision-making process.

Another unique aspect is that social care has to be delivered against a range of national minimum standards or benchmarks. These set out to define what is *minimally* acceptable for the ways in which services are delivered and their aims and objectives. An organisation that does this exceptionally well or is able to 'go the extra mile' would take us some way to delivering a 'quality' service. Further, any definition of quality must incorporate the views of both service users and service providers. To be effective in this, such an organisation must have a reliable and robust system in which it can assess and understand the needs and expectations of its service users. This may involve developing internal processes (between departments, teams or colleagues) and external processes (involving other agencies, providers or suppliers) to make this happen effectively. Martin and Henderson have referred to this as the *quality chain* (2001, p180).

A quality service in social care

Moullin's categories (2003) attempt to define the key features of a quality service. We can build on these in order to define what specific features are unique to developing a quality service in social care. This may lead us to create a more detailed list as follows.

- The importance of providing services capable of meeting the exact needs of service users/carers.

- Services easy to access or obtain, in the right place, at the right time, and at the right level.

- Equality in access and provision regardless of social, ethnic or cultural background.

- Reliability, consistency and continuity.

- Services that have a clear purpose and rationale contained within a statement of its aims and objectives and a description of the minimum standards or level that people could expect.

- Services that are in keeping with the legislative framework.

- Services provided within the costs and resources available but which are efficient, effective and give value for money.

- Being delivered by people who are committed and competent and who receive good quality training, supervision and support to do the best job possible.

- Services that are socially acceptable, inclusive and involve service users/carers in their design, delivery and evaluation.

Further, Adams (2002) reminds us that the application of quality (and quality assurance) to social work practice is inevitably deeply enmeshed in the politics of its management. He reiterates that regulation in particular can be a double-edged sword. On the one hand, accountability through service standards and the registration and inspection of the workforce can be empowering for service users, but on the other hand the bureaucratic nature of this process can 'swamp' professionals and stifle creativity (p287).

What is quality assurance?

As discussed earlier, a full appreciation of how to improve the quality of public services is hampered by conceptual problems and a confusing terminology which is inconsistently used (Ring, 2001). 'Quality assurance' (QA) is a commonly-used term which originated from manufacturing in the 1980s but has now been widely adopted by the public sector. A range of techniques related to QA has since been developed including statistical process control, quality circles, total quality management and the use of model systems such as those developed by the British Standards Institute (www.bsi.org.uk). We will return to look at some of these techniques later. However, it is only in the last decade that concerted efforts have been made to apply QA to health and social care in the UK.

The term 'quality assurance' is often used interchangeably with 'quality control'. The latter describes activities and techniques employed to achieve and maintain the quality of a service, but in itself contributes only one step towards QA. Quality control essentially involves monitoring activities that can detect and eliminate any causes of poor quality. Therefore quality control is the process through which organisations measure actual quality performance, comparing it with the standards set and then acting on the difference.

Adams (2002, p288) identifies this *rectification of errors and shortcomings, maintenance through standard-setting, enhancement through audits and evaluation and quality maximisation* as one of the main approaches to quality used in social care. This has been well illustrated by the frequent use of (public) inquiries and investigations as a key means of translating remedies into practice. Managing quality to achieve excellence in social care services through quality assurance, on the other hand, requires a more holistic approach to management within an organisation. This entails establishing a system focused on achieving quality: assessing its adequacy, auditing how it operates and reviewing the system itself. In a quality assurance system, the search for excellence is ideally driven from within the organisation rather than being imposed from the outside. This is supposed to incorporate a never-ending improvement cycle to ensure that an organisation learns from its results, systematically standardises and documents what it does well, and improves the way it operates and what it delivers, all from what it learns (www.dti.org.uk).

In essence, quality assurance systems promote the notion of getting it right first time, of self-audit and of avoiding wasted effort and inappropriate behaviour (Patel, 1994).

> *Quality assurance is the measurement of the actual level of the service provided plus the efforts to modify when necessary the provision of these services in the light of the results of the measurement.* (Williamson, 1979, p631)

Therefore, a quality assurance system entails taking a planned, systematic and conscientious approach to creating a climate and culture of quality and excellence that permeates the whole organisation.

The very nature of social care services and the unpredictable and turbulent environments in which some organisations operate however do not always enable them to fall in neatly with traditional models of QA systems. Later on we will explore how these ideals and principles can become compromised or may conflict with external social, economic and political pressures on an organisation's performance. Similarly, systems that focus on more scientific or quantifiable measures as the main means of evaluating the effectiveness of services or 'products' can lack meaning where the 'human services' are concerned. For example, measurements of the outcomes of interventions which are focused on 'quality-of-life' may be more congruent with social work values and practice and could play an important part in measuring quality in any systems being designed and implemented (Felton, 2005). This is illustrated in the case study below.

CASE STUDY

Exploring the link in individual planning for people with learning disabilities between quality of planning and quality of life

Person-centred planning is a key initiative central to the vision of Valuing People (DoH, 2001b) but this has been criticised for the lack of evidence-base underpinning its implementation as a widespread policy initiative (Rudkin and Rowe, 1999). Plans are seen as a paper exercise in which individual goals are not translated into the daily programme of support to people using services. Adams et al. (2006) explored the extent to which individual plans enhance the quality of life for people with an intellectual disability by comparing the plans and outcomes for people from residential settings using a goal rating scale and direct observation. They found few relationships

between having a 'good' individual plan and the actual outcomes in terms of quality of life and concluded that training on how to provide support to people in pursuit of goals on their individual plans would be at least as important as training in the individual planning process itself. They did however reveal a trend towards those users with plans that were prepared to a higher quality in that they tended to spend more time engaged in meaningful activity as a result. This was particularly significant where staff were supported to do so or that organisational factors like management direction were present and contributed particularly in areas thought to improve the quality of life for service users such as increasing community presence and community participation.
(Source: Adams et al., 1999)

Quality management systems

Before going further, I would just like to mention other quality frameworks that you may come across if working in the various organisational environments within which social care services are delivered. Within the NHS, clinical governance provides the overall framework for continuous quality improvement, although this framework does not prescribe in any detail how service quality is to be secured. The Commission for Health Improvement (2002) defines clinical governance as a *system of steps and procedures . . . to ensure patients receive the highest quality care.* The aims of clinical governance are: to raise patient satisfaction; improve collaborative relationships and efficiency within and across clinical teams; increase job satisfaction for professionals; improve clinical outcomes and reduce significant events (Gerada and Cullen, 2004). Governance is often viewed as a multi-layered and complex concept. At its simplest, however, it can be described as the way in which organisations and the people working in them relate to each other. A review of governance and incentive structures that help influence health care organisations to be more responsive to change (DoH and SDO, 2006) found that more work needs to be done to build a learning culture for new governance and incentives to improve care. Given the complexity of relationships within governance, increased collaboration between researchers, practitioners, government and service users is recommended to deepen understanding of their world views and priorities.

For those working in or in partnerships with local authorities, Best Value is another means by which local authorities are expected to account for the quality and responsiveness of services and this will continue to be the instrument for improvement in public provision at the local level (DETR, 1998). Best Value is not specifically a quality management programme but is a government initiative which replaced compulsory competitive tendering. Within Best Value, each service is systematically and continuously reviewed in order to focus on promoting better standards and demonstrating quality and value for money. The emphasis is on working actively in partnership and with greater flexibility with the independent sector so that both quality and costs are taken into account when awarding contracts. Best Value has a service user/citizen focus and an emphasis on continuous improvement, value for money and performance measurement (Moullin, 2003). Within multi-professional service environments such as Trusts for mental health or learning disability services, there may be more flexibility about how different quality assurance systems are utilised. Alternatively a systemic approach to improving service quality may be more difficult to achieve in these circumstances.

Key components of a quality assurance system

Now we have defined what we mean by quality assurance, we will go on to look at the three key components of any quality assurance system. These can be identified as:

- **a focus on the customer** and whether the service gives its customers what they want, as measured by outcomes for service users, e.g. satisfaction surveys or representation and complaints procedures;

- **understanding the process** through the design and operation of the service process to use resources in the most efficient way to meet service user requirements;

- **professional quality** by ensuring that all employees are committed to quality and excellence by working within professional procedures and standards.

In the subsequent chapters of this book, we are going to look in more detail at perspectives on developing outcomes for service users and their participation and involvement in the process. We will also be examining the central role of workforce development as an essential aspect of quality management. For the remainder of this chapter, therefore, we are going to focus on understanding the process, i.e. how one might design and operationalise specific aspects of a quality assurance system.

Quality assurance systems – Donabedian's model

In 1969 Donabedian divided the evaluation of quality of care into the evaluation of the *structure* in which care is delivered, the *process* of care and the *outcome* of care. His findings are still highly valued, forming the basis of much current work on quality assurance in health and social care. These are equally dependent on establishing standards, as underpinning standards in any quality assurance system are crucial to Donabedian's analysis and go some way to providing valid and acceptable definitions of what we mean by quality. The existence of standards, either nationally- or locally-determined also helps to identify what specific criteria are needed in order to measure and evaluate performance against standards in terms of effectiveness and quality (Sale, 2000).

Donabedian's model is one which picks up on the interrelated 'quality' elements; for example, structural inputs, process relationships and service outcomes. These are all essential to each other in order to achieve quality in the final outcome. The process of achieving this is equally important which Donabedian (1980) explains as follows.

- **Structure** – this incorporates the stable characteristics or organisational frameworks within which care and support are provided. Staffing arrangements, financial resources, management roles and hierarchy all contribute to the overall structure of an organisation. The stability or instability of structure can increase or decrease the probability of good organisational performance, by the way it aids planning, or the design and implementation of systems. In summary, stable structures and organisations provide stable bases for the continuous monitoring and evaluation of service delivery.

- **Process** – the interaction and relationships between practitioners and service users are essential to incorporating and transferring values and ethical principles during the delivery of care. The presence of professional autonomy and service user participation would be examples of this. These factors are important to ensure that the design, delivery and evaluation of care and support services are firmly embedded in the organisational policies, procedures and practice to which the core principles of equality, diversity and holistic approaches are demonstrable.

- **Outcomes** – defined as the changes resulting from, or attributed to, the service provided. These include social and psychological as well as physical aspects of performance.

ACTIVITY **2.2**

You are asked to consider the first element, that of structure as identified by Donabedian. How does the structure of your organisation impact on your own particular team or service area? What threats or opportunities can you identify in examining the different characteristics of your organisational structure – for example, staff and financial resources, the process of restructuring and change, hierarchies of management control? How might these contribute to or undermine your local system for monitoring quality in the services you currently provide?

Donabedian's latter elements, process and outcomes, are directly related to the legislation and policy guidelines in social care that prioritise the philosophy and practice of listening to service users (Mitchell and Sloper, 2003), as we shall see in Chapter 4 later. Despite theoretical models and research findings, there is still a gulf between theoretical ideals and actually achieving these indicators in the everyday experiences of service users and their networks, as well as finding ways to express these in quality assurance systems (Carr, 2004). People who use services have stated that they want the following things.

- A proper assessment of their individual needs – this should be the starting point for commissioners.

- Care that is needs-led, not service-led, recognising that different people have different needs.

- Care that is provided to meet the needs of people, that a person is 'not just a number'.

- Continuity – services should change only if and when a person's needs change.

- Services provided by people and organisations that genuinely understand the people who use them – the importance of user-led organisations should not be under-estimated.

- Services that allow people to be spontaneous, to do what they want, when they want.

- Services that empower people and allow them to exercise choice and control over their lives. (Commission for Social Care Inspection, 2006, p9)

A preoccupation on the part of many organisations with structures and processes rather than outcomes for users/carers means that barriers to change persist. Commissioning systems set up specifically to meet quality standards can perversely focus principally on inputs rather than on outcomes for people. This affects their capacity to evaluate need and be flexible and innovative in their response. This is one of the most profound challenges facing both commissioners and providers of social care services, particularly where quality is concerned.

CASE STUDY

The use of individualised budgets to personalise social care towards more outcome-based support in West Sussex

Individualised budgets are an initiative stemming from the Health and Social Care White Paper (DoH, 2006a). One of the English pilot sites has enabled a person needing care to do an assessment of their own needs, often through a web-based tool. The services they need are then worked out through a resource allocation system (RAS) and a system of support brokerage. Once the council has confirmed an individual's choices, people can then construct their own care package and choose a range of services that bear no relation to the traditional 'menu' by designing their own circle of support using leisure, transport, health and financial services as well as social care. As a senior manager from West Sussex put it, 'If what people choose is not what councils offer, councils and independent providers may not survive – the lesson is change or die'. (Source: CSCI, 2006)

Whilst the types of approaches described above are not yet the norm for people using social care services, they raise even wider issues about assuring the quality and safety of those services which are purchased by individuals, as well as more traditional organisations, and the validity of people's choices when public money ceases to be public. The key point here is that the importance of involving service users in decisions about what constitutes quality and value for money is an active consideration at every level and is likely to become a greater imperative in the future if government plans for models of service delivery are to be realised.

The use of national standards and national standard frameworks

The need to be able to formulate and apply standards of quality is not only internal to particular organisations and individuals but is universal to the whole system of care. In Chapter 1 we referred to national service frameworks (NSFs) which attempt to spell out basic standards for all the different service user groups which are based on research evidence (DoH, 2001a). The introduction of national minimum standards over the last decade has established different sets of standards for different care services, including statutory, private and voluntary, plus hospitals and nursing agencies in England. The content of NSFs and their implementation involve extensive analysis of the quality of care that must be provided by specific services. NSFs are defined in a way that enables them to be measured by using indicators of quality and performance or by identifying shortfalls in provision.

Earlier on we identified the key characteristics of a service standard. When managing services, setting clear standards can help to assess the level of service you are providing and communicate expectations by making explicit what professionals do – it is important to understand where standards, either national or local, fit into the quality assurance cycle. When devising and writing your own standards it is helpful to start by working backwards, looking at what you want to achieve and using outcome criteria. Outcome criteria are descriptive statements of the performance, behaviours or circumstances that represent a satisfactory, positive or excellent state of affairs. A criterion is a variable selected as a relevant indicator of the quality of care and must be measurable, specific, relevant, clearly understandable, clearly and simply stated, achievable, professionally sound and reflective of all aspects of those it is applied to, taking into account their physiological, psychological and social circumstances. Outcomes can be measured using both quantitative and qualitative measurements and these measurements are required at both the individual and the service level.

Performance indicators are therefore just one aspect of measuring outcomes and when combined with more qualititative measures or research, such data can powerfully illuminate aspects of professional practice or measurement (Tilbury, 2004). The case study below illustrates one of the performance indicators used to reflect progress on one of the national standards within children's services.

CASE STUDY

National performance indicator no CF/D35 – long term stability of children looked after

Within the Every Child Matters *(2003) outcomes framework, one of the indicators designed by the government under the umbrella broad outcome 'staying safe' is said to help illustrate and measure the relative effectiveness of councils in achieving longer-term stability for children looked after (CLA). For those CLA for as long as four years, it is stated within the standards on which this indicator is based, that it reasonable to expect that a substantial amount of that time is spent with the same foster carers or that an adoptive placement would be made. Stability and the opportunity to develop and sustain strong attachments are fundamental in terms of improving outcomes for looked-after children, particularly those who spend a considerable period of time in care. Performance against this indicator is also related to the achievement of the government's national public service agreement target for looked-after children to narrow the gap in educational achievement between looked-after children and their peers as stability and educational support are seen as linked. For your information, the average performance in England of children perceived to be 'stable' within this indicator has been 50% with virtually little change within the last five years. (Source: CSCI and the National Statistics Office, 2005b)*

The question of what should be counted, and the extent to which indicators are supported by research findings, are both important if they are to have credibility in assessing effectiveness. According to Tilbury (2004) the availability of data may shape how performance is conceptualised and what *can* be counted rather than what *should* be counted (p234). As illustrated in the indicator above, the focus of most child welfare data-sets is on outputs (amount of service provided or number of clients served) which is one of the reasons why it is difficult to measure outcomes where there is little routinely recorded data. Tilbury (2004) reminds us, however, that counting something can also highlight its importance in resource and practice terms. In the example given above we would want to know more about the quality of the care the child receives, its cultural appropriateness and about other factors that promote security for children. These are important aspects of the stability of the placement albeit they are not so easy to measure or evaluate. A single indicator reflecting the time spent in a single placement cannot safely be viewed in isolation, as it inevitably emphasises quantity over quality and is not necessarily a true measure of stability and security. Output data, however, does have a place in highlighting patterns of service delivery and bringing to the forefront questions about how power may be allocated to certain policy positions where one indicator is selected to evaluate certain aspects of child welfare over others.

The provision of family support services also lies at the very heart of the debate about the relationship between the state, parents and children. A lack of attention to this aspect in the conceptualisation and implementation of performance measurement, according to Tilbury (2004), can reinforce those very practices that seek to diagnose, rescue and treat without improving child safety or family wellbeing. Performance or outcome data therefore have to include other dimensions such as process, effectiveness and efficiency, and should be used in conjunction with other methods of evaluating and developing services such as research, inspection and financial modelling, as well as being linked to quality and performance improvement strategies (p234).

Whilst I have taken quite a simple approach to making this point, I would like to leave you with the question (based on the above discussion) of what other outcome criteria you would use to measure stability for children looked after. You may also like to consider what skills and knowledge you and your staff would also need in order to do so. In addition to having an understanding of the subject matter itself, designing an outcome measure may require skills and knowledge in information systems, information technology, process mapping, statistical skills and research methods (Pinnock and Dimmock, 2003), in addition to specialist skills that might be needed to engage with this particular service user group. Martin and Kettner (1996) have suggested six criteria for judging outcome measures, which are: the *utility* of information so that it is useful and relevant; the *validity* of indicators to ensure that they are actually measuring what they claim to; definitions on which an indicator is based to ensure *reliability* and *consistency* in interpretation; the *feasibility* of data collection in a way that it does not interfere with direct work with service users or breach data protection; and finally, the *cost* of data collection where we need to ensure that collecting information does not outweigh the benefit and is the most effective way of doing so. Martin and Kettner (1996, cited in Pinnock and Dimmock, 2003) also discuss the importance of putting outcome measures to practical use, for example, in comparing one outcome with another as a benchmark or as a feature of unit-costing.

In this last section we have been discussing how we must recognise within any quality assurance cycle the importance of conceptual models of evaluation before we can fully appreciate any meaning behind the measures or indicators we are being asked to use. The quality assurance cycle involves establishing firstly the philosophy of care, which requires our consulting and confirming beliefs about service users' support and care needs. These are further underpinned by professional codes of practice, as well as moral beliefs in turn underpinned by relevant legislation – for example, human rights and not least the values and principles held. As a manager or leader of quality, and in order to evaluate the quality of your service, you need primarily to be able to describe your service in measurable terms. Those involved should be able to articulate exactly what they do and the reasons why they do it in a certain way. Based on all of these, you should be able to identify appropriate standards and criteria for evaluation and think about which models might be useful; for example, Donabedian's structure, process and outcomes framework. Sale (2000) recommends developing a measurement system with suitable tools to facilitate the collection of data using both a retrospective and current audit, so that when these are collated, they will give a fuller picture of the quality of services delivered.

One of the challenges in setting national standards is that the multiplicity of different standards for service provision in agencies cannot always be reconciled with the principle that all service users should have equal access to services of an equivalent quality which meets their needs. Where there is discretion, the variation in services offered will not always be ideal (Adams, 2002). This is one of the drivers behind star rating systems and league tables in performance management. For example, returning to the case study on the measurement of long-term stability for CLA, variation in performance across providers is a particular concern in fostering services, given the variation in unit costs of placements between independent and council-run agencies. On average, agencies in the private or voluntary sector met 77 per cent of standards, whilst council agencies met 72 per cent (CSCI, 2005b). Although not a major difference, at least some of the differences in fees may be attributable to a better quality service. There is still more geographic variation in the performance of council agencies, as in the period 2004–2005, 27 out of 146 council agencies failed to meet half the required standards for child placements and three met less than one quarter. The overall picture therefore suggests that children's chances of a good quality placement still vary across the country (CSCI, 2005b, p120).

ACTIVITY 2.3

Before going on to look at more holistic system approaches to quality assurance, I would like you to think about your own service area, and identify one area where you think there is a need for a local service standard. One example might be the provision of induction for new staff in your service. Use the following questions to help you think through your own role and the roles of others in implementing a local service standard.

ACTIVITY **2.3** *continued*

- *How do you go about designing, recording and publishing a standard for your service?*
- *What is the difference between a standard and a policy and a procedure?*
- *Where does your standard fit in with evidence-based practice?*
- *How would you monitor or evaluate the outcomes from implementing your standard and what sort of measures might be appropriate?*

Total quality management systems

Earlier in this chapter we looked at the differences between quality control and quality assurance, both of which are important aspects of quality management. Total Quality Management (TQM) builds on quality assurance, but consciously extends to addressing the management, people and issues involved in achieving lasting quality improvement.

The difference between quality management and TQM is that the latter involves working with partner organisations to ensure quality for its service users throughout an entire organisation rather than just in one area. TQM requires everything to be integrated to ensure quality throughout an organisation and as an ongoing process it demands commitment from the top, involving everyone in an organisation to meet the requirements of services users and other stakeholders whilst keeping costs to a minimum (Department of Trade and Industry, undated). Ideally, all the members of an organisation feel part of, and have ownership in, the various levels of the organisation (strategic, operational, customer and development).

The task of implementing TQM can be daunting, since to be able to become a total quality organisation, bad practices must also be recognised and engaged with. A lack of direction or leadership may result in firefighting or reactive behaviour, or individual services and departments working in isolation. Whilst TQM must involve everyone, to be successful it must start at the top with the leaders of an organisation, who must provide a well-developed mission statement followed by a strategy which can be translated into action plans throughout the organisation. This involves skills in leadership and in understanding the culture of an organisation, using that knowledge to successfully foster teamwork and cooperation at all levels (we will be looking at these aspects more closely in Chapter 3). The building blocks of TQM are mainly concerned with the quality of the processes used to translate inputs (e.g. referrals, resources, equipment and training) within an organisation into outputs (e.g. services, information or products). Within TQM, processes provide the fundamental building blocks of all organisations and the steps by which we add value. Therefore processes need to be continuously redesigned and reviewed to make sure that an organisation is able to continue to improve – to rethink, restructure and streamline the business structures, processes, methods of working, management systems and external relationships by which we create and deliver value (Talwar, 1993).

For example, in social care, it is imperative that the number of process improvement activities undertaken is matched by an organisation's ability to resource and implement these without harmful disruption to day-to-day delivery of services. Initiative-overload and fatigue can be a common problem in the care sector and ultimately counterproductive. Councils, for example, face a number of challenges in how they manage their resources so that they can make services more person-centred and deliver the government's future agenda. Increasing people's choices alongside the agency's ability to widen its portfolio of services is by no means cost neutral. In adults' services, for example, councils are finding it difficult to manage the shift from an historical profile of services to one that embraces a wider range of alternatives. This includes the development of domiciliary care – preventive and simple services that might play a part in promoting and maintaining people's independence and well-being (CSCI, 2005b, p186).

Such wholesale shifts, irrespective of pilots and other research, undoubtedly require transitional resources from central government. Making the most of process management within the TQM model may focus particularly on economic development services and on external partnerships to find ways of redesigning services through joint commissioning and procurements. According to the theory of TQM, whereas the outputs of an organisation go to its 'external customers', i.e. service users and carers, the outputs of the internal processes of an organisation go to 'internal customers', i.e. the staff. If the needs and expectations of each internal and external customer are consistently met or exceeded, then these can be said to have achieved 'total quality'.

So far we have looked at a number of ideas and concepts in relation to quality, and it may strike you that an implementation framework is needed to build on these and pull them together to achieve organisational excellence. The Excellence Model described below attempts to do this, based on many years of research, education and advisory work at the European Centre for Business Excellence (www.dit.gov.uk).

Excellence models

The Excellence Model was launched by the European Foundation for Quality Management (EFQM) in April 1999. It is an approach to quality that enables organisations to assess themselves against a set of criteria for excellence, and to use this self-assessment to do two things: to identify which areas need to be improved and to consider how best to bring about the changes needed. 'Excellence' in this model is defined as outstanding practice in terms of the core service and how it is managed, delivered and – more to the point – viewed by the people who use it (Walker et al., 2003). The Excellence Model also recognises that processes are the means by which an organisation harnesses and releases the talents of its people to produce results. These are thus the 'enablers' who produce the 'results'.

Assessment against enabler and results criteria is normally a team activity, giving a score based on identified strengths and improvement opportunities leading to action planning. Approaches to self-assessment can use a number of different methodologies. Organisations can also gauge their achievements by applying for many of the quality awards in Europe or the UK.

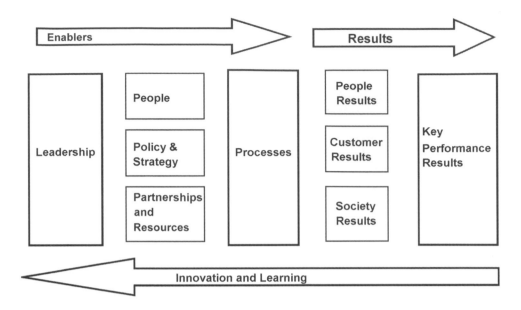

Figure 2.1 *The EFQM Excellence Model*

The Excellence Model consists of nine elements:

- Leadership: how leaders develop and help the organisation towards excellence.

- People management: how the organisation supports its workforce.

- Policy and strategy: how the organisation plans its activities to ensure continuous improvement.

- Partnerships and resources: how the organisation plans and manages its external partnerships and internal resources.

- Processes: how the organisation manages and monitors its activities.

- People results: what the organisation is achieving in relation to its staff.

- Customer results: what the organisation is achieving in terms of the people who use its services.

- Impact on society: what the organisation is achieving in relation to the expectations of the community.

- Key performance results: what the organisation is achieving in relation to its planned performance. (Department of Trade and Industry: www.dti.gov.uk/ quality/excellence)

Obviously there are limits to how far one manager, practitioner or team can go to systematically and critically review the quality of services offered within their organisation as a whole. In our next chapter, we will be looking more closely at what can be achieved through teamwork within your area of responsibility and generally how as an individual you might understand and contribute towards the culture for quality improvement. The activity below is designed to help you think about the first steps required in a more concrete way.

The relationship between quality and costs

Poor quality services are inevitably associated with a variety costs. These can be product failure costs, i.e. the costs of discarding or under-using poor quality goods and services, or process failure costs, i.e. where there has been an inefficient use of materials or human resources in the process. In social care, these may manifest themselves as unnecessary bureaucracy, poor quality communication and the inefficient use of resources. The costs associated with poor quality are not just financial but may also result in time-consuming complaints, legal issues, or the need to provide additional or compensatory services. The public reputation of an organisation and its staff will also be inevitably damaged by poor quality services, not to mention the impact on users/ carers and the community, as evidenced by research documenting longer-term problems resulting from poor quality interventions with looked-after children or for adults living in institutions.

The question of quality and costs in relation to prevention provides further challenges – for example, how far can public sector systems recommend the resourcing of new and additional services where there is still unmet need? Or, how can we judge whether services are being delivered at prices that potential and existing service users and carers can afford? The case study below illustrates one example of such a dilemma, demonstrating that the careful monitoring of quality improvements from all perspectives needs to be implemented.

leaving hospital, to increase their long-term chances of independence, or for those at short-term risk in order to avoid further hospital admissions and can be provided in a range of alternative settings.

Common practice has been to provide intensive short-term rehabilitation placements in nursing homes (Steiner, 2001). Jacobs and Rummery (2002) conducted a study of nursing homes in England and their capacity to provide rehabilitation and intermediate care services. They found that while the quality of nursing care offered by nursing homes was an important determinant of successful intermediate care, support by local NHS services, in particular rehabilitation using physiotherapy, speech, language and occupational therapy, was in short supply and their capacity to provide additional support to nursing homes to maximise recovery appeared unrealistic.

In such situations, nursing homes purchased these services from private providers or employed their own staff. Jacobs and Rummery (2002) found that these additional costs were reflected in the fees charged to residents. Self-financing older people found themselves subsidising the costs of health care for publicly funded residents. Jacobs and Rummery recommended that for local commissioners to be successful with intermediate care placements in nursing homes, consideration should be given not only to the quality of care offered by those homes but also to commissioners' own responsibilities for funding or providing health care and equipment. Otherwise, these placements will serve only to shunt the problem of 'bed-blocking' into the independent sector and will not restore the functional independence of older people as intended.

Limitations of quality assurance systems and quality management

This chapter will conclude by summarising some of the limitations of quality management. The main criticism of quality assurance systems is that by and large they are designed by civil servants, policy makers and senior management teams in the public services, in a direction often dictated by politicians (Adams, 2002). This situation has the potential to provide a battleground between managerial and professional interests and values where top-down quality assurance techniques adopted by government, local authorities and their partners and managers in social care may not achieve the objective of guaranteeing the quality of services when they conflict in some fundamental ways with the more empowering goals of social work. Selecting and developing outcomes and indicators of quality are subjective processes and ultimately contain implicit values about what is important in practice and how best to intervene and provide support to service users and carers, their networks and the community.

We will see in Chapters 4 and 5 that the discourse on quality and performance measurement can be understood within broader debates about service user involvement and evidence-based practice and how our increasing knowledge and participation in these areas of practice can impact on policy-making and our knowledge about what makes a quality service. The relationship between our actions and what we know about their impact is important in building further the knowledge base in social work and social care, and how the measurement of both quality and performance can be used politically, economically and organisationally to shape the future direction of social care. As Tilbury (2004) put it:

> *performance measurement is part of the policy process and attention is required to the political and economic context in which indicators are developed and used. Management objectives such as value for money cannot be assessed without reference to good practice. Secondly, indicators do not provide uncontested facts about performance, but represent concepts and ideas that can permeate policy debates.* (p228)

Therefore assumptions and values about what is good practice are embedded in indicators and these must be uncovered and analysed.

CASE STUDY

Using inspection reports and care plans to plan service improvement

Watson (2004) examined the issues for front-line workers within nine residential childcare units, giving their feelings on how recent government-sponsored quality enhancement initiatives have impacted on service delivery. A central component of the planning process for young people in care is through individual care plans which have become increasing related to the concept of quality enhancement and the attempt to achieve specified outcomes for young people in care. In units operating successfully, care planning appeared to be integrated into the daily work of unit staff by using the plans as a working tool for day-to-day decisions made in relation to individual young people. These decisions were then discussed at staff meetings to consider progress and to set goals for the foreseeable future. As a result the practice moved from a reactive to a more proactive and consistent approach in their dealings with individual young people so that a culture was created as a result of the effective utilisation of care plans.

In units which were seen to be struggling, care plans were more likely to be completed as an administrative task, but not as part of the ongoing process of actually responding to or working with the young people. Care plans in these units were perceived as tasks which the agency could check and subsequently hold staff accountable for and their lack of impact on practice was also affected by pressure of work and the reactive nature of such units. In effect, care planning became a tool or paper exercise that met the requirements of the organisation, but at best merely touched on the real work of staff.

In relation to inspection, Watson (2004) looked at how inspection reports were used to develop and enhance the level of quality. He found that reports provided strength in relation to a unit's bargaining/negotiating position with external managers to improve specific aspects of the service, so that it was not so much the standards but the recommendations of the reports that became important to unit staff. External managers were found to over-emphasise tangible issues at the expense of

CASE STUDY *continued*

developmental and practice activities and unit heads found themselves having to spend considerable time on administrative tasks at the expense of working with staff to improve the quality of the service.

The study concluded that developing quality was much more complex than defining and measuring performance and then expecting front-line service providers to respond to this activity. The notion of empowerment of front-line workers was affected by the notion of accountability. Watson recommended that to develop a quality culture and service strategies for enhancement required looking at how these actually apply within specific sites, services and power relationships which start from service providers experiences.

C H A P T E R   S U M M A R Y

In this chapter we have surveyed the literature on quality and considered its relevance or usefulness for our purposes in social care. Evaluation of quality in social care can take place at various levels. At a national level, there is a number of charters and accreditation bodies which set standards for care services and at this level, organisations are measured against pre-set standards or external set criteria. At the purchasing level, standards are specified within a contract with set indicators. At the provider level, it begins to become more complex when we start to deal with the people involved in delivering the service.

Whilst measurement of quality provides useful tools, ultimately improvements in quality require changes – including changing the way things are done, changes in processes and changes in the behaviour of people and teams of people. Whether a quality improvement programme encompasses an entire organisation with a major change, or whether a team of people reorganises into a single service on a smaller scale to improve it, then the same principles of change-management apply. Potential areas for improvement in commissioning and organisational practice have been suggested here, all of which have resource implications if social care is to realise its full potential in maintaining and providing quality services.

In the next four chapters we are going to look at some of the more practical implications of developing a quality service through developing a culture for improvement, service user participation and the use of evidence-based practice to link staff knowledge and skills in improving services. All of these areas are important aspects of an organisational development to manage quality and performance.

FURTHER READING

Shaw, I, Greene, J and Mark, M (2006) *Handbook of evaluation: policy, programme and practice*. London: Sage.

Provides a useful reference for any practitioner or student interested in examining the complexities of contemporary evaluation and the ongoing dialogue that arises in professional efforts to evaluate people, services, policies and practices.

Commission for Social Care Inspection (2005b) *The state of social care in England 2004–05*. Using the performance assessment framework, this provides an overview and summary of what the current issues and challenges are for social care. (Available from **www.csci.org.uk/publications**)

Department of Trade and Industry
Provides a range of literature on its 'From quality to excellence' page. (**www.dti.gov.uk/quality**)

Chapter 3
Leading and managing a culture for improvement

Introduction

The previous chapter looked at some of the 'harder' or more tangible aspects or characteristics of organisations that deliver quality services, and touched on the systems and resources required. We will now go on to look at less tangible aspects of organisations that are considered crucial to achieving quality, for example, concepts of organisational culture and leadership. Academic literature on organisational culture has tended to assert a relationship between strong unified cultures and commercial success particularly where quality and performance are concerned (Clegg et al., 2005).

To explore this relationship further but in the context of social care, this chapter will draw on theories of organisational and workplace culture and the central role that leadership is thought to play in managing cultural change in order for quality improvements to be successfully implemented. Growing interest in organisational culture lies in the recognition that this is an important factor in achieving organisational effectiveness. A key challenge for managers, therefore, is how they might understand, monitor and actively manage the culture of their organisations (Davis, 1984). This is certainly not an easy task, but you can begin by developing an awareness, understanding and insight into the history of your organisation, as well as the key events or contexts that have helped to shape its identity (Schein, 1992). Developing your own leadership skills and the leadership skills of people in your service area is also thought to be an important source of influence on organisational culture, and essential to leading and facilitating a team approach to developing quality services.

We will begin this chapter by examining the concept of organisational culture and by identifying what factors to look out for within the workplace that contribute towards a healthy environment in which quality services can develop and thrive. We will then go on to examine leadership theory, the differences between leadership and management and the role of leadership in promoting quality care. Towards the end of this chapter, you will be encouraged to develop an agenda for local action by identifying areas in your particular service where there is a need for quality improvement and how you might engage your team members in this process. We will expand on concepts such as team working, partnership, motivation and delegation.

What is organisational culture?

There has been a continuous growth of research into organisational culture which has sought to study certain aspects of an organisation, such as its climate and its human resource management. This is combined with an increasing recognition that achieving change cannot be achieved by just focusing on structural reform and the systems of an organisation, or by emphasising the different variables and roles in the workplace that emphasise efficiency and management to improve performance. This could, perhaps, explain why public organisations are facing pressures to adopt management techniques utilised by the private sector. We need, however, to be aware of the limitations of the managerialist perspective when talking about the feasibility of managed culture change. Davis (1984) and Brown (1998) argue for tapping the potential offered by studying organisational culture. They propose that this provides a non-mechanistic, more flexible and imaginative approach to understanding how organisations work.

Much of the research into organisational culture has taken place in commercial organisations, although within the management of health care there has been a move to capitalise on this area to improve patient care (DoH, 2000c, 2005a). Within social care, the promotion of concepts such as 'learning organisations' has outlined the value of positive cultures as an important ingredient in the way organisations evolve and learn (SCIE, 2004; Gould, 2000). The complexity of this area is reflected in the lack of consensus as to how define 'culture', as every aspect of an organisation is in fact a part of its culture and cannot be understood as separate from it. Many aspects of culture are intangible and difficult to see. Buono et al. (1985) talk about it being multi-dimensional and concerned with traditions, shared beliefs and expectations of organisational life which include ways in which people interact with each other, perform their work and even their dress code, all of which are powerful determinants of individual and group behaviour (p482). Gordon (1991) observes that an organisation's culture is a product of successful adaptation to the environment and is to a significant degree *an internal reaction to external imperatives* (p404).

Conventionally, organisational culture literature is divided into two broad streams. One approaches culture as an attribute or something that exists within an organisation, alongside structure and strategy. The second regards culture more globally by defining the whole character and experience of organisational life for which culture is a metaphor. The distinction between the two has important policy implications (Scott et al., 2003) in terms of whether, like other attributes, culture is capable of being manipulated to satisfy organisational objectives and as a means of re-engineering an organisation's value system. By contrast, in taking a systems approach culture becomes the defining context by which the meaning of organisational attributes is revealed. For the purposes of this chapter, however, we will tread a middle path between these two approaches. We will not assume that culture is controllable but our aim is to try and appreciate its main characteristics so that we can at least describe and assess these to help us think about how this impacts on our own objectives to provide better quality services.

The linking of quality to issues of organisational culture can be observed from investigations into high-profile enquiries in social care which have highlighted cultural problems as key factors contributing to critical incidents or failures (Cooper, 2005). Research has also shown the importance of culture in contributing towards high quality outcomes for service users and carers (Gould, 2000). We have already identified that tremendous pressures to adapt to significant changes in the external environment are embodied in the constant political, social and economic upheavals for social care organisations, many of which have then to restructure or reinvent themselves in order to respond and to bring about change. As highlighted earlier, whilst structural reforms are important and necessary, they are not capable of delivering their intended impact without also giving equal attention to influencing organisational culture. The ultimate success of these structural reforms depends also on the acknowledgement of the psychological and social aspects of an organisation that influence how people think, what they see as important, how they behave and how they support the organisation's mission (Cameron and Quinn, 1999; Hafford-Letchfield, 2006b).

The different faces of organisational culture

Every organisation has four cultures; the one that is written down, the one that most people believe exists, the one that people wished existed and finally, the one that the organisation really needs. (NHS Chief Executive, cited in DoH, 2005a, p1)

As we go through this chapter you will be asked to think about your own local culture, mostly within your immediate team. It is important, however, to recognise that the culture can vary at different levels and so the task for managers trying to promote a healthy culture is complicated by the potential for conflict arising from multiple stakeholders, each of whom will have their own agenda or vision and be working from a different perspective and with a different set of criteria or expectations. Observation suggests that few large and complex organisations are likely to be characterised by a single dominant culture. This does not necessarily mean that this would result in a better performance than in an organisation with pluralistic cultures. Where organisations are not differentiated along clear occupational lines, such as in modern multi-professional teams, there will be a number of co-existing subcultures. According to Scott et al. (2003), subcultures may share a common orientation and similar espoused values, but there may also be disparate subcultures that clash or maintain an uneasy symbiosis.

Classifications of subcultures

Complex organisations, such as care trusts or national charities with local providers can be characterised as comprising a variety of co-existing subcultures. Scott et al. (2003) identify three types of sub-cultures vis à vis their organisational functionality.

- **Enhancing cultures**: these represent an organisational enclave in which members hold core values that are more fervent than and amplify the dominant culture. For example, specialist or expert teams which constitute centres of excellence.

- **Orthogonal cultures**: an organisational enclave which tacitly accepts the dominant culture of the organisation whilst simultaneously espousing its own professional values, for example NHS clinicians within a Care Trust who maintain allegiance to the Royal Colleges.

- **Counter cultures**: an organisational enclave that espouses values which directly challenge the dominant culture. For example, resistance by specialists or disciplines to broader management diktats or to the limitations of professional freedom as a result of increased management of care.

Implied within the above is something about the 'unwritten rules' within an organisation. Unwritten rules form one of the most powerful ingredients of culture (DoH, 2005a) and are described as such because they are not often openly discussed in meetings or in formal documents and this absence of discussion or infrequency of debate can lead to rules being rarely questioned or challenged. Further, unwritten rules are usually shared by most, if not all, the members who work in a team and provide a common way for everyone to make sense of what is going on around them, to see situations and events in similar ways and to behave accordingly. All of these factors combine to have a powerful influence on how people behave at work, often without them realising it.

ACTIVITY 3.1

Based on what you have read so far, what evidence of 'the culture' exists in your own team or service area? Is this positive or negative or are you unsure? You may want to consider such issues as the level of trust within your team, the clarity of communication and the systems used, whether the roles of team members are clearly defined. How often, for example, are innovations expressed and capitalised on in your team? How often does conflict surface and what mechanisms exist for resolving conflict? Finally, how interested are members in developing their knowledge and skills and how are these encouraged and supported?

In relation to your own role within your team or service's culture, take some time to think about your own sense of satisfaction, emotions and feelings of competence at work. How do these feelings impact on your team and the day-to-day work within it?

Being overwhelmed by trying to work out which expectations and practices are required within a team or service can take up a lot of energy. Cultural differences between departments or services within an organisation can be striking and do little to ensure quality in services where there are so many disparities and a lack of clarity. It is natural for most people working in social care not to want to change their location, style or mode of working and they will not embrace or engage with plans for changes which, to them, do not obviously link to improvements. In these situations there will be resistance, as the case study below illustrates.

CASE STUDY

When Adefolake joined 'Visions' as a new manager, the community development service for people with physical disabilities, she found morale and commitment to the work very poor. This was manifest in a number of administrative systems, meeting schedules and patterns of service delivery that had not changed significantly in three years. Individual members of the team tended to bypass management in their day-to-day work and Ade's attempt to try and pin down everybody's roles and responsibilities was extremely difficult.

During supervision, Ade found a number of individual staff very negative about the service and expressing a desire to leave their jobs. There had been a couple of new national and local initiatives that had been well resourced in order to improve social inclusion for service users, but staff in 'Visions' were not capitalising on these or engaging with the wider agenda, resulting in little impact by initiatives on the overall service. Ade became of the opinion that the service lacked vision and that there was a lack of mutual trust between senior managers and staff in the department.

The culture within any organisation or team must support the direction of change by rewarding behaviours which support it and move towards an environment in which a team can learn and where problems are approached in an integrated way. Johnson (1989) identified various elements that contribute to organisational culture and which influence change; for example, he talks about *formal and invisible power structures*, the latter developing to enable people to bypass formal procedures for decision-making and to hold informal or invisible power which can be used to block change. In the case study above, whilst Ade has authority in her new role as a manager, the lack of clarity about the roles and responsibilities of staff in her service does not permit her to use her power and authority to lead without really making this authority visible. Reiterating and making explicit the formal structure of work in the service and its relationship with the overall *organisational structure* (Johnson, 1989) will also help to clarify the different levels of responsibility and establish the direction of the service. The formal structure may have to change in order to achieve a transformation in the way work is done. Ade may find that 'Visions' is in competition with staff in another part of the organisation or externally, and these issues need to be identified together with any opportunities to work together to integrate and improve services. Resistance to change often reflects a lack of trust and needs to be overcome through careful listening and explanation to reduce misunderstanding.

Johnson (1989) also talks about an organisation's *control systems* and adapting control systems to accommodate any new ways of working. Within 'Visions', the administrative systems and meeting schedules will need to be reviewed and resource systems such as finances, information and staffing will have to be examined to establish how these support proposed service changes or not. Current *routines* within the work, both formal and informal, will need to be scrutinised so that poor practice is challenged and addressed and good practice is encouraged and rewarded. Spelling these out into policies and procedures in ways which involve staff as far as possible will help to clarify specific roles and responsibilities. Moving toward a culture of learning supported by improved communication and training for those involved will also help them recognise that change does not always follow a rational, linear pattern of decision-making such as that spelt out in service objectives at a more strategic level. Organisational policies and actions must reinforce what is communicated and behaviour must match the rhetoric.

At times of tension, it can be helpful for managers to involve different people in building a shared vision. This requires both leadership and good management skills in order to constantly demonstrate both the desired direction of change for improvement and also to illustrate that managers mean and do what they say. Enabling participation in any changes also takes time and requires skilled leadership (as we will see below), which implies paying attention to the development of the participants' skills as well as the evolution and practice of leadership characteristics in managers themselves. Good quality management and staff learning can ensure that managers provide support for their colleagues and find new ways of working and learning together. The attention to workforce development in social work and social care since 2000 (TOPSS, 1999) recognises that a team will have its own culture if the people working in it have been together long enough to experience significant challenges together, have been trained and have developed and, together, embraced diversity in both staff and service users.

Leadership theory and the role of leadership in promoting quality care

Leadership is often cited as the key to improving quality and organisational performance which by implication makes the development of leadership within organisations critical. There are many theories and definitions about leadership as well as substantial research on how 'do' it, despite which there remains much uncertainty about what is required to be an effective leader (Bass, 1990; Kotter, 1990; Higgs, 2003). You can study leadership from a variety of perspectives, including the different traits, behaviours and situations that inform leadership theories and the development of such concepts as transformational (Bass, 1990), charismatic and transactional leadership (Clegg, et al., 2005).

Leadership development is open to everybody working in organisations providing social care and is often based on relationships that occur within the leadership situation in response to particular issues or challenges. For example, a leadership role might be taken by a person progressing an improvement or change in response to legislation or feedback from service users/carers and this builds on the recognition of their expertise, experience or interests, as well as the need to drive or implement significant change. This makes leadership more context specific or situational (Barker,

1997). Underlying this notion is the view that leadership is all about being able to adapt and be flexible to ever-changing situations and contexts. You cannot study leadership without focusing on the interactions between those who lead and those who follow, or by not taking account of followers' perceptions (Yukl ,1989).

Adair (1983) believed that a leader must balance three very wide and different needs in approaching a task: the needs of the task itself; the needs of the group or team working on the task; and the needs of the individuals within the group. Attention to detail within all three aspects helps leaders to structure a more thorough approach to a new situation. The contribution of contingency leadership theories transfers easily to the social care arena. These take into account the context of leading and the nature of the work being led. Contingency theories also consider the internal working environment and the external economic and social environment (House, 1995). Many organisational theorists interested in leadership also refer to the inherent political nature of the work environment which requires the acquisition of 'political skills' to help people like managers in social care to become more adept at using their interpersonal and information management skills to more positive effect (Ahearn et al., 2004).

Political skills are defined as the ability to effectively understand others at work, and to use such knowledge to influence others to act in ways that enhance one's personal and/or organisational objectives. By being political, managers work through others, developing effective networking and alliances. Managers or leaders who operate in this way are thought to be in a better position to secure resources for their teams and become more valued by them (House, 1995). This accumulation of friendships, connections and alliances allows managers to leverage their *social capital* to facilitate change within a climate that encourages learning for service improvement (Hafford-Letchfield, 2006a; Hafford-Letchfield et al., 2007).

Distributed or dispersed leadership

Modernist and postmodernist leadership theories have proposed that leadership is a socially constructed concept (Boje and Dennehey, 1999) and that in social care, therefore, substitutes for leadership can be found instead in one's professional experiences. Those professionals who possess a high level of expertise may be one or several members of your team, who might be involved in decision-making, goal-setting, performance measurement and evaluation, and will take responsibility for determining how these issues are progressed. It is thought that in situations where there are high levels of trust, shared responsibilities, interdependence and support, leadership can be substituted by the process of empowering staff and allowing steps to be taken to address the power inequality inherent in subordination as based on principles of mutual respect and supported autonomy. This requires, in turn, empowered managers who can motivate individuals and teams to achieve more towards organisational objectives by granting them greater independence from managerial control.

As we have seen throughout the book so far, this is not an easy concept to address within the care sector where legislative and regulatory responsibilities take precedence. Dispersed or distributed leadership may, however, be an aspiration that you adopt for your team or service area, where tasks and goals are shared and based on a common framework of values and where members work together to pool their expertise. Distributed leadership therefore *concentrates on engaging expertise wherever it exists within the organisation rather than seeking this only through formal position or role* (Harris, 2003, p14) and is largely equated with team working and collaboration which contribute towards an ideal culture for learning. It is strongly influenced by the professional cultures and subcultures which shape a practitioner's identity, and the organisational or department cultures in which the team is situated (Eraut, 2006) is often enacted as a distribution of responsibilities to meet operational needs rather than as an aspiration to the distribution of power in itself.

Since the people in the workplace and the relationship with service users both play such important roles in the leadership/management equation in social care, their understanding of these terms and their conceptualisation of leadership are vitally important (Kotterman, 2006). In the next chapter we will be considering the leadership role played by service users themselves through approaches that promote user participation and the active role that the service user movement has played in strategic developments. Service users' own feedback has highlighted the importance of leaders and managers knowing how to *show the way, keep people on board and together, listen to customers, make change happen and get results through the best use of people, money and other resources* (Skills for Care, 2004a, p1). In summary then, many of these principles are embodied in the social care leadership and management standards (Skills for Care, 2006) and the GSCC codes of practice (www.gscc.org.uk). Good social care managers are said to possess distinctive qualities and are those who:

- inspire staff;
- promote and meet service aims, objectives and goals;
- develop joint working/partnerships that are purposeful;
- ensure equality for staff and service users which is driven from the top down;
- challenge discrimination and harassment in employment practice and service delivery;
- empower staff and service users to develop services people want;
- value people, and recognise and actively develop potential;
- develop and maintain awareness and keep in touch with service users and staff;
- provide an environment and the time in which to develop reflective practice;
- take responsibility for the continuing professional development of self and others;
- demonstrate an ability to plan organisational strategies for workforce development. (Skills for Care, 2004a)

Leadership and management

So far we haven't distinguished any differences between leadership and management, as we have been working under the assumption that the value base of care provision gives some impetus to a paradigm shift towards distributed leadership and increased participation, which in turn influence a culture for improvement. However, managers who are leaders themselves are important in achieving this ideal. Conceptualising and defining the differences between leadership and management are not straightforward, as the two terms are often used interchangeably both in the workplace and in the management development literature on social care (Skills for Care, 2004a). Researchers hypothesise that if effective workplace management represents some combination of leadership and management, the approach used by effective managers to accomplish objectives must be significantly different from that of ineffective managers, but both have profound and important effects on those they manage (Yukl, 1989).

Both leadership and management roles may have an involvement in establishing direction, aligning resources and motivating people. Managers, however, are thought to be more focused on planning and budgeting, while leaders establish direction. Managers have been perceived as having a much narrower purpose, by trying to maintain order, stabilise work, organise resources and become the arbiter of quality standards (Kearney, 2004) where predictability and order reign. Leaders, on the other hand, are said to be those who produce the potential for dramatic change, chaos, and even failure (Kotter, 1990).

Leadership styles can vary – for example transactional leaders will implement a series of exchanges between themselves and followers and this is perhaps closest to what we understand about management. Transactional managers pay attention to all the necessary and critical management functions, such as clarifying roles and tasks and allocating work through the exchange of rewards and sanctions (commonly known as the 'carrot and the stick' approach). Transactional leaders also adhere to organisational policies, values and vision and are strong on planning, resource management and meeting schedules, but may not cope so well with major change or managing the change process.

Charismatic leaders, alternatively, create the impetus for change and are said to have strong interpersonal skills and the ability to create a grand and idealised vision. Charismatic leadership often emerges in times of crisis and is found in settings that are characterised by opportunity and optimism, where they unify people towards a vision and foster conditions of high trust (Clegg et al., 2005). Transformational leaders are those who are often seen as being opposite to transactional leaders because they deal mostly with abstract and intangible concepts like vision and change. Key factors in successful transformational leadership have been identified as a concern for others, approachability, integrity, charisma, intellectual ability and the ability to communicate, set direction and manage change (Clegg et al., 2005).

Gardner (1990) wrote that the term 'manager' often suggests an individual who holds a directive post in an organisation, a person who organises functions, allocates resources, and makes the best use of people, and Gardner contrasts what he calls the *leader manager* and the *routine manager*. The leader manager is concerned with thinking longer term, developing an organisational vision, reaching longer-term goals and values and motivating others. The routine manager is more strongly associated with the organisational structure, s/he thinks and acts in the shorter term, accepting and maintaining the status quo (Bass, 1990; Gardner, 1990). Nebeker and Tatum (2002) suggest that management involves continuously planning, organising, supervising and controlling resources to achieve organisational goals. Planning is associated with providing what the customer wants and developing a way to provide it. Organising and supervising involve developing an organisational structure, reward systems, and a performance management system. Controlling encompasses measuring processes and product characteristics, sustaining production processes, reducing variation, providing customer satisfaction, and anticipating short-term needs. Managers take responsibility for those processes and are constantly seeking to improve them. Leaders on the other hand, are looking to the future in anticipation of their organisation's global needs and long-term existence (Kotterman, 2006).

The key roles, skills, competencies and attitudes defined by Skills for Care (2004a) have attempted to combine what is needed to be both an inspiring leader and a professional manager in a large and complex environment where both roles are even more difficult to assimilate in one person. Too often, senior managers believe they are leading when in fact they are managing and quality assurance may be one area which is typically over-managed and under-led. Managers are expected to demonstrate leadership qualities through leading by example or heading up a project or initiative, whilst still performing the functions of management. Schein (1992) identified what he termed *culture embedding mechanisms* which can be used to try and change the culture and climate of a department. These were:

- what leaders pay attention to, measure and control on a regular basis;
- how leaders react to critical incidents and organisational crises;
- observed criteria by which leaders allocate scarce resources;
- deliberate role modelling, teaching and coaching;
- observed criteria by which leaders allocate rewards and status;
- observed criteria by which leaders recruit, select, promote, retire and excommunicate organisational members.

In summary, a leader of quality improvement needs all of these skills and more. In the words of Trice and Beyer

> *Managerial practices are probably the most potent carriers of cultural meaning. As the proverb says, 'Actions speak louder than words'.* (1993, p365)

Using emotional intelligence to promote successful teams

The concept of emotional intelligence has been frequently applied to the field of leadership where Goleman (1996) claimed that in order to be a successful leader, the presence of emotional intelligence far outweighed either IQ or technical knowledge. Within the differing theories about emotional intelligence, Goleman's (1998) definition is the widest ranging and the most performance orientated, encompassing abilities beyond the specific processing of emotions, including self-awareness, emotional resilience, motivation and drivers, empathy and sensitivity, influence and rapport, intuitiveness in relation to decision making and conscientiousness. Emotional intelligence is not an end in itself but an important component of thinking and action in order to facilitate quality service delivery and outcomes. In relation to organisational culture, the importance of emotion has been described as a central organising system responsible for the coordination of behavioural, psychological, affective and cognitive responses to major adaptive problems (Panskepp, 2000, cited in Morrison, 2007). Morrison (2007) makes the point that *emotional responsiveness and capacity are not merely a product of individuals, but are powerfully influenced by collective and contextual processes, including workplace, professional and social cultural factors* (p253).

Within the collaborative nature of care, the ability to work cooperatively with colleagues, supervisors and other agencies is further complicated by the organisational and inter-agency context. Menzies (1970) identified the presence of social defence systems which are unconsciously reflected in organisational rituals, process and systems designed to avoid feelings and experiences that are too deep and dangerous to confront. Thus problematic micro-level interactions between staff often act out unspoken macro-levels tensions within and between organisations. Leaders with emotional intelligence can help to reduce any inter-group hostility, and encourage difference. Further, as Morrison (2007) reminds us, where values and knowledge about discriminatory forces are integrated with inter-personal skills, particularly within multidisciplinary settings, staff are enabled to work across boundaries more effectively. In short, the ability of both managers and staff to be aware of both resonant and dissonant emotions allows them to be more able to manage these and also to be more anti-discriminatory in their roles (p258).

Effective teams: a symptom of healthy leadership

Many traditional approaches to effective teamwork tend to view teams as an approach to getting the job done. However, arguments have been made that effective teams are not goals in themselves within an organisation, but are the result and culmination of healthy leadership (Crother-Laurin, 2006).

Organisational transformation does not begin with management providing or mandating opportunities for collaboration or teamwork, but starts instead with individuals in an environment where leaders foster the learning and development of these individuals so that collectively the organisation can rely on the capacity and contribution of each member. One of the challenges currently facing the social care workforce is the ability to attract, develop and retain talented employees who can work effectively and efficiently together. Management and leadership development which includes diversity and succession planning can also contribute to staff 'buying in' to the vision being promoted (Hafford-Letchfield and Chick, 2006c). Staff who trust their managers are those who are told that their relationships are important and that connections, interdependencies, and integration are at the heart of their organisation.

In Chapter 2, the key quality systems that we looked at which have evolved out of the quality movement included attention to the process i.e. relationships, networks, inter-dependencies, teams where there are integrated and holistic approaches, synergy and connections. In short, there is a recognition that the relationships between people and processes are more valuable than anything which management theory can offer us. People who have low control over their work and working environment are hurt physi-cally and emotionally (Pine and Healy, 2007). According to Crother-Laurin (2006) there must be an infrastructure in place to invite any opportunities to work as a team and foundational thinking that guides the infrastructure, which begins with the thinking involved behind the action. Systems thinking (such as we saw in the Excellence model in Chapter 2) is therefore quite an important aspect of leadership development, parti-cularly in relation to difficult types of problem-solving where an inherent dependence on others or the past helps to identify the root causes of problems.

Senge (1990) has identified systems thinking as the foundation stone for the develop-ment of learning organisations and for fostering effective teams. Argyris (1993) has also influenced thinking about the relationship of people within organisations, collective learning and action research. He discovered that conflict tended to exist between indi-vidual personalities and the organisational management structure. The tendency for managers to exert power over people at lower levels of the organisational hierarchy produces fear, passivity and ambivalence which are all in conflict with the key principles of leadership in social care. Given the difficult context of social care management where crises often occur and resources are frequently stretched, the theme of participatory management – where professional social work and social care staff are empowered to make decisions about the job and on the job – cannot be underestimated.

Using learning to enhance cultural awareness and promote improvement

Evidence supporting the value of learning in the context of promoting cultural change can be found in a variety of sources (Schraeder et al., 2004; Hafford-Letchfield et al., 2007) and is essential to the success of such initiatives as TQM in bringing about changes in the norms, values and certain structures within an organisation. We will therefore be looking more closely at the use of staff learning and development stra-tegies in Chapter 6 and how this should be built on evidence-informed approaches to practice in Chapter 5.

Managers have a significant role to play in facilitating the learning and development of staff and can aim to develop their confidence by leading learning forums with them. Using opportunities at team development days, meetings with a developmental focus can give staff a chance to work through real or hypothetical exercises which are closely related to their own specific situation to try and find solutions to recurrent problems. Using these situations to work with groups to develop some recommended alternatives for the organisation, and even where participants are encouraged to prepare these in the role of senior managers or service users, should be the bread and butter of a manager's role. This experience can expose participants to some of the thought processes, rationale and challenges associated with the need for a similar cultural change in their own organisation, or allow them to realise that the changes taking place are necessary for the long-term survival of the organisation beyond surface level assumptions.

ACTIVITY 3.2

Identifying and developing areas for improvement in your own service area

We have been discussing some of the less tangible but theorised aspects of developing a culture for improvement. You might wish to now turn to the list of questions below which are designed to help you focus on aspects of your team which may help or hinder any planned service improvement. You can use these 'storming' activities here to consider in more detail how you might go about leading any improvements to your service and you can then use your thoughts or notes generated from the following areas of questioning to plan for an initiative within your own service area that currently needs attention.

First of all, think about the change in your service that you wish to make. It can help to break this down into a SMART objective (Specific, Measurable, Achievable, Realistic, Timely). When you have identified this you can use the following questions (adapted from DoH, 2005a) to develop a participatory management strategy.

Q.1 Am I the right person to lead this improvement?
Consider the context, your skills and influence. What further skills and knowledge might you need to develop if you don't have these at the moment? Do you need to develop your leadership skills or are there others in your team who can take a leadership role? What incentives might there be?

Q.2 Is my team keen to be involved in this improvement?
Early engagement of key team members is important in the successful spread of new and sustainable practice. Teams who identify a desire to be involved rather than being directed to do so, and who already have an interest in improvement, will really help. Using team development opportunities to engage the team may be a useful first step as front-line practice staff will have a lot to say about those issues they face on a day-to-day basis and may relish the opportunity to air these constructively.

Q.3 What evidence is there of interprofessional and collaborative working relationships?
The active engagement of other professionals, either internally or externally, in your service improvement will promote its chances for success. This includes all the professional, managerial and support staff, as well as those people from other agencies. How can you engage other significant professionals in your action plan? What forums are available to share concerns and ideas? Who might you link up with to forge a working partnership?

Q.4 What support have I got from my own manager?

Even if they are not taking the leadership role, managing upwards and the participation of senior staff in your service improvement are equally important. Improving performance has to relate to the objectives of the wider organisation and any local business plans so that these are made meaningful at a team level.

Q.5 Can I allocate any dedicated or protected time for the team and significant individuals involved to meet, liaise and undertake the improvement activities?

Dedicated time set aside for regular meetings to review current practice, to plan and evaluate service improvements is certainly required. There are many tools you can use to kick-start the process, for example appreciative inquiry which is a form of action research that attempts to create new theories, ideas or images that assist in the developmental change of a system (Cooperrider et al., 2003). It is a method used to promote cooperative searching for the best in people and their organisations by the practice of asking questions that strengthen a system's capacity to heighten positive potential. Appreciative inquiry is also based on the principles of equality of voice, where everybody involved is asked to speak about their vision for the service or changes they wish to make. Traditional approaches to change look for the problem, make a diagnosis, and find a solution. The primary focus is on what is wrong or broken, since we look for the problems and through the process emphasise and amplify them. As an alternative, appreciative inquiry suggests that we look for what works in an organisation. The tangible result of the inquiry process is a series of statements that describe where the team/organisation wants to be, based on the pinnacle moments of where they have been already. Because the statements are grounded in real experience and history, people know how to repeat their success (Hammond, 1998, p6–7).

Q.6 Are there any anticipated additional demands or changes relating to this service?

Many improvement projects have not been sustained or implemented easily owing to unforeseen pressures and competing demands or priorities. These should be minimised if possible or alternatives considered. You should start an improvement project only if there is a realistic opportunity of taking it forward, otherwise you run the risk of initiative-fatigue or overloading staff and draining their enthusiasm.

Q.7 Will the team identify this as a high priority and will they also recognise the priorities of other services and work towards joint solutions where there is conflict or competing demands?

Priorities may differ between managers and staff, and between departments, services or organisations. A recognition of these potentially competing agendas and a commitment to work cooperatively where these exist are required for sustainable change. There must also be a willingness to learn from mistakes if the improvement is not successful. Learning from mistakes can be a feature of reflective management and practitioners, if they are willing to be accountable and take responsibility for professional decision making.

ACTIVITY 3.2 *continued*

Q.8 Will the team integrate this initiative within normal working practice such as incorporating job descriptions, policies and protocols? Does the team recognise this as a long-term commitment rather than a short-term project?
Sustainable change needs to be embedded within normal working practice. Short-term thinking which considers improvement as a 'project' with an end point will cause problems for sustainability. Embarking on sustainable change will inevitably involve risk-taking. You should also be willing to acknowledge success, no matter how small, to re-motivate and energise staff. Staff will need to be given time and resources on the basis that they will use these to develop further.

Q.9 Is there a commitment to, and available resources for, the collection of data relating to the benefits of the improvement?
To encourage others to adopt new practices and also to ensure sustained improvement, it is important that all benefits of the change initiative can be demonstrated. It is therefore essential that there is an understanding of the need to collect and use evidence and data and that there is an effective support/infrastructure in place for this, such as IT systems, skilled staff, etc.
Source: Building and Nurturing an Improvement Culture. DOH 2005a

Resistance to planned culture change

Trying to develop a culture of improvement can be challenging, particularly in complex environments. Given that organisational culture is transmitted via a wide range of media including established working procedures and practices, it is unrealistic to expect culture-change strategies to be effective on all these fronts simultaneously. This requires realistic timeframes to implement the multi-level changes required; for example longer-term strategies such as those laid out in *Every Child Matters* (DfES, 2003) span a proposed ten-year programme of reform. According to Scott et al. (2003), key sources of organisational inertia and resistance include a lack of ownership, as changes often evokes a sense of loss. Reaction to changes by individuals or professional groups can be negative and unpredictable and can disrupt the best laid plans. The influence of external factors can also sometimes work against internal reform and may involve external stakeholders who have conflicting priorities to your own. Leadership plays a central role in any cultural transformation and so the lack of it will result in resistance. You may need to think about how to integrate the different styles of leadership; i.e. transactional, which is based around securing organisational compliance and control by using material motivational factors, or transformational, which inspires cognitive change by redefining the meaning of information to which organisational members are exposed (Scott, et al., 2003, p115).

To achieve cultural change there needs to be a belief in the potential for leadership, not only by the manager but also by staff and service users, and an atmosphere of trust and honesty where personal and professional development is actively encouraged, valued and supported. Earlier on we touched on staff commitment which has been found to be greater among staff with higher job satisfaction and more job control (McLean, 2002). Not surprisingly, McLean found that receiving contradictory instructions, having responsibility without power, feeling overwhelmed with users' problems and disagreement over good practice affected all workers' commitment. Being able to make a difference to users' lives and being part of a team, however, definitely increased job satisfaction. Therefore, inclusion and involvement are important components of commitment, suggesting that a supportive workplace is one way of avoiding excessive stress. In summary, an improvement culture will be one where all these aspects are present, shared and lived by the people in the team or service.

C H A P T E R   S U M M A R Y

Social care organisations are facing incredible pressure to adjust and evolve to meet the demands of both the government and the public to deliver improved quality services which are often under-resourced. These demands will likely necessitate changes in the culture of your organisation and this chapter has discussed how the examples of leadership and teamwork can promote change by also giving attention to the culture and ethos within which change can be managed. Whilst the culture of an organisation is constantly evolving, it is important to note that fundamentally changing an organisation's culture is actually a much longer-term endeavour (Schraeder et al., 2004). It is important for leaders to recognise that changing an organisation's culture to improve quality may evoke strong emotional reactions from employees. Providing them with the foundations to support changes in the culture, by setting an example through ethical management and your own leadership skills, can have a profound influence on their willingness to support or resist change. Allowing employees to participate and become involved in making the changes in their culture through facilitating their own leadership skills can have a profound impact on their willingness to buy-in to the changes (Schraeder et al., 2004, p502). Regardless of the approach taken, leaders should remember that communication plays a powerful role.

The feasibility of cultural change in social care is contested terrain, but nevertheless is an important factor to take into account when considering how to develop quality improvements. Many of you will have enough direct influence on your local area of practice to develop one of the subcultures in which this can thrive. The crucial role of leadership and being aware of common barriers and tools that can be used within teams and services will help you generate the culture required. The qualities of a leader manager include the ability to articulate the bigger picture; encourage team members to work to their strengths; to protect the team from to inappropriate pressure and to represent them up and down the hierarchy, as well as external to the organisation. Leader managers use authority and power appropriately; explicitly focus on service users; interpret the changing political context; allow time to explore and articulate concerns, ideas, information and discussion to encourage ownership; and; have a commitment to maximising the skills, knowledge and resources of the team. Finally leader managers possess an emotionally intelligent approach, where staff are given good quality feedback, coupled with a good personal manner, respect and reliability. To be successful, teams have to explain and solve the various challenges that come their way, and if these work well enough they will build up the expertise and confidence to deal with future challenges so that this starts to become part of the team culture. It follows, therefore, that a team will have its own culture if people in the team have been together long enough to have experienced challenges together (we will look more closely at the relevance of recruitment and retention to this notion in Chapter 6).

Studies of interprofessional team cultures highlight characteristics that can account for professional differences within a sector or team (Cameron et al., 2000) and can disrupt a service on the basis of status, prestige, knowledge, language, focus, orientation and time perspectives (Huntington, 1981). This will present managers with the task of providing as many opportunities as possible to help staff understand and resolve problems together and to observe the impact of this on their team and their service.

FURTHER
READING

Martin, V (2003) *Leading change in health and social care*. London: Routledge.
This provides an overview of leadership theories and a practical guide to management tools and techniques. It assumes no previous knowledge of change management and shows that leaders can and do emerge from all areas of service provision, that leadership is shared and collaborative and not the sole responsibility of senior staff.

The NHS Modernisation Agency
(Has provided a number of *Improvement Leader's Guides* which can be downloaded from **www.modern.nhs.uk**
There are six guides to choose from:
• Improvement knowledge and skills
• Managing the human dimensions of change
• Building and nurturing an improvement culture
• Working with groups
• Evaluating improvement
• Leading improvement.

Appreciative Inquiry Commons (2006).
Available online at **appreciativeinquiry.case.edu**

Chapter 4

Managing outcomes for service users and the role of service users as arbiters of quality assurance

Introduction

Within the UK context, service user participation, or user involvement as it is now often referred to, has become a cornerstone of social care and social work policy and philosophy. People's expectations of social care services are now a significant driver of the way in which services are commissioned and provided. There is also a legal requirement for user involvement within adult and child care, and family policy and practice, as well as in the community as a whole. This reflects the broader agenda in public policy. For example, the White Paper *Our health, our care, our say* (DOH, 2006a) states that people who use or require social care support are a fundamental resource in their own care and in determining the formulation of policy and service developments. Although we are clearly a long way from achieving this vision, the involvement of those who use services is an increasingly important way of evaluating quality. The emphasis on a consumerist agenda, which we referred to in Chapter 1, came from increasing custo-mer choice and consumer involvement in a mixed economy of care, based on a political and ideological shift towards the market and the purchase of services. This is under-pinned by the idea that if service users' requirements are identified then service providers can offer a more efficient and economic service. New Labour's 'Third Way' expressed the political commitment to public participation in politics, via the devolu-tion of local government, user involvement in public services, the human and civil rights of disabled people and combating social inclusion (Beresford and Croft, 2001). The democratic approach to service user involvement is primarily concerned with empowerment and the redistribution of power, and with people gaining more control over their lives (Begum, 2006).

Whichever approach is taken, arrangements for participation now permeate all new partnerships across public provision, from health to housing to education, and with a particular emphasis on public involvement in regeneration policy. In successful organisations, service user involvement sits close to corporate decision-making bodies and is represented on those bodies which help to oversee service user involvement and plans. Some commentators (Beresford and Croft, 2001) have argued, however, that user participation in social work and social care has predominantly been based on the consumerist agenda, relying more on methods that are bureaucratic and managerially and professionally driven. This development, they suggest, is not always successful in increasing personal and political power and ultimately the empowerment of service users, but in many ways control of the system still remains with the service or organisation.

It is implied here that user participation is in danger of becoming a means to an end rather than an end in itself, an outcome which we should seek to avoid. Using participation as an essential tool to improve social care should promote a democratic approach emerging from service users' rights and requirements. Any participation strategies have to include more practical ways to base participation on the direct experiences and perspectives of service users and their representative organisations.

As this book is about quality, we will be focusing specifically on the role of service users in enhancing quality and continuous improvement by thinking through the different ways that we can meaningfully involve them. The needs and expectations of people who use social care services should drive changes in the way services are commissioned and delivered (CSCI, 2006), thereby making it a priority to find out what people want and need, and to involve them in how services can be developed – based on their lived experiences, rather than on organisational systems and processes as illustrated above. Particular care needs to be taken to reach those people who have complex needs and/or difficulty in expressing their needs.

This chapter aims to look at some of the practical ways in which service user involvement, participation and control of social care services can enhance quality and continuous improvement. We will start by identifying the key principles of service user involvement using evidence from the service user movement itself. We will define what we mean by the terms 'participation' and 'outcomes' when talking about service users and carers and will look at the evidence for improving social care services through participation. We will then identify any barriers to successfully achieving this. We will conclude this chapter by identifying methods by which managers of local services can improve accountability, transparency and openness in order to have an impact on service quality, practice and outcomes. For the sake of clarity, within this chapter we will be talking about services users rather than carers. Many of the issues raised are also relevant to the participation of carers, who provide essential support and plug many of the gaps in social care as well as offering valuable insights and perspectives. However, as carers may also require social care support themselves, in this respect, they are service users in their own right (Begum 2006) and shall be referred to as such.

Defining participation

Participation and user involvement have become common currency where the two terms are used interchangeably in an imprecise way. For the sake of simplicity, Begum (2006) regards user involvement as a component of participation where users of services participate in decisions that affect their lives at an individual level. At a collective level, this includes participation in decision-making, policy formulation, service development and in the running and controlling of services (Begum, 2006, p 3). Wright et al. (2006) remind us that participation is not an isolated activity, but a *process* by which service users are empowered and supported to influence change, either within an organisation or by directly leading in policy and service development. There are various models spelling out the different levels or stages of relationships between service users and providers (King's Fund, 1992) with different focuses, such as citizen or consumer, and different intensities of users' interaction with the state (Politt, 2003), as well as hierarchies of involvement such as those illustrated in Arnstein's Ladder (1969). Arnstein's model emerged from citizen involvement in planning in the USA. Each rung of the ladder represents the degree of power a citizen holds, making a fundamental point that participation without a redistribution of power is an empty and frustrating process. This allows power holders to claim that all sides were considered, but makes it possible for only some of those sides to benefit and to maintain the status quo. Suffice it to say, in all models setting participation out in this way there is no assumed progress from one level to another, as this depends on the situation or the validity of the different levels of participation at different stages of policy and service development. There is, however, widespread agreement at both a national and local level that all levels of participation are nevertheless important and worthwhile (Begum, 2006).

As we saw in Chapter 2, there are various aspects to quality in public services and a number of different groups with something to say about how it should be defined. Because there is this range of interested parties, forms of participation and involvement in the public sector are quite different from those in the private sector (Pfeffer and Coote, 1991). Cowden and Singh (2007) differentiate between two opposing discourses about the user movement; one in which users' successes, particularly in the arenas of disability and mental health, have given them a voice in decision-making, research and education; the other where progressive critiques have been incorporated into a managerial system, moving the agenda away from ways in which users' rights might be developed and expanded, to an agenda of how users can advise on how to best 'target' existing or diminishing resources. The overall limit to available resources is certainly one important issue that affects the extent to which all those who could be involved in decision making actually are. Another crucial issue is the question of power. Without defining the context in which this can be addressed, the voice of the user becomes what Cowden and Singh refer to as a 'fetish', *something which can be held up as a representative of authenticity and truth, but which at the same time has no real influence over decision-making* (2007, p16). These are harsh but very real criticisms for managers and practitioners who genuinely wish to make progress in this area. We will start our discussion of how this might be achieved by focusing on broader objectives for participation in relation to the concept of outcomes-based care.

Outcome-based support and care

Outcomes are the changes, benefits or other effects that happen as a result of an organisation's activities (Charities Evaluation Service, 2006). Outcomes can be physical, psychological or social. They can be as much to do with achieving a better quality of life, such as users getting involved in employment and/or developing healthy relationships with people close to them, as it is about receiving a particular service or range of services. Adopting an outcomes approach means planning and managing the work so as to bring about particular outcomes – and then finding out what outcomes, intended or unintended, you are actually achieving. Much of the research conducted around outcomes and quality has examined the experiences of various groups of users of community care services. We can distinguish between aspirations that are associated with particular circumstances, such those associated with using a particular service, and those which relate to the broader concept of quality of life. Within the research about users' experiences of services common themes often arise, such as the importance of retaining independence and autonomy, being in control of how one lives and having one's priorities respected (Harding, 1997). Prerequisites for maintaining independence and keeping control may also include financial security, appropriate and timely information, and keeping a healthy body and mind (Henwood and Waddington, 1998).

Researchers who have looked at outcome definition by different groups of service users have found a powerful consensus that links their views (Qureshi and Henwood, 2000). This is illustrated in a statement made by *Shaping Our Lives,* a project funded by the Department of Health from 1997 as part of the Community Care Development Programme. The project established a National User Group, bringing together people with physical and sensory impairments, older people, people with learning disabilities and users/survivors of mental health services.

> *We want to be empowered as citizens and members of society and to achieve meaningful equality. Meaningful equality means having the same choices, opportunities, rights and responsibilities as all other members of society. It includes being able to live independently with the support that we require as a result of our impairments. Being empowered and independent means having full choice and control over the way we live. It is particularly important in relation to the provision of support services.* (DoH, 1997)

As we will see in the next chapter, the emphasis on outcomes is driven by an evidence-based approach to policy and practice and draws a distinction between quality of life outcomes and service process outcomes (Qureshi et al., 1998). The experience of receiving a service has a number of other impacts on service users which also reflect its quality. For example, Qureshi and Henwood (2000) talk about the way in which services are delivered as well as the way in which someone tries to access services.

Users of social care services have argued that the way in which something is done can completely undermine the value of achieving some of the quality of life outcomes that are more commonly promoted. Qureshi et al. (1998) have coined the term 'service process outcomes' to describe these impacts on the process of service delivery. To illustrate this, Henwood and Waddington (1998) explored the perceptions of older people using domiciliary care services. Judgements about service quality were typically a reflection of two components: the nature of the relationship between the user and the carer or support worker, and the way in which care was delivered. A quality domiciliary care service, they found, was characterised by the following features.

- Staff reliability.

- Continuity of care and staff.

- Kindness and understanding of care workers.

- Cheerfulness and demeanour of care staff.

- Competence in undertaking specific tasks.

- Flexibility to respond to changing needs and requirements.

- Knowledge and experience of the needs and wishes of the service user.

These attributes can be seen as likely to contribute to both the attainment of process outcomes and the quality of life outcomes. Taking these on board cautions against an over-concentration on developing and using those standards relating only to organisational activities, at the expense of exploring the extent to which quality can be individualised. This may of course not be true for all service users and there will be important differences in rankings between different groups, specifically in relation to age, gender, ethnicity, sexual identity and so on, and within different levels of service use. Qureshi et al., (1998) argue that a possible way forward to improve quality might be to ask service users themselves whether they had any preferences or priorities which related to the way in which services were delivered. The task would be to then try and implement these, rather than deliver punctuality or continuity of staff to everyone. With finite resources available, an over-concentration on providing services that meet certain quality standards, without reference to the importance of these dimensions to individuals, may limit the capacity of services to respond flexibly to individual requirements. Qureshi and Henwood (2000) suggest, therefore, that service users may be prepared to 'trade-off' different aspects of quality which would allow them greater control over what is most important to them.

Service user involvement for quality care – key principles

Commitment to participation should be visible in the principles held and the practices demonstrated by senior management teams. These can then be built into the departmental or agency values and reflected in strategic planning, delivery, resourcing, communication and business improvement activities. Commitment to participation should extend to staff development activities where opportunities are provided to enable staff to develop the skills and attitudes to engage effectively with service users and carers as part of their everyday work. Some hierarchical agency structures may make participation a challenge in some settings (Henderson and Seden, 2004). It is important in these situations to avoid tokenism where participation doesn't really fit with the short-term results orientation of the organisation. Even in these circumstances, Pine and Healy (2007) assert that it is never efficient to reach a decision that no one will implement or commit to due to a lack of involvement (which here includes both users and staff). Thus, even with a medium-range perspective on efficiency, participation can often strengthen programme implementation and successful service outcomes (p54). This is evidenced in the case study later on where two different models of quality assurance approaches used in a mental health day services had very different outcomes. The first approach did not involve services users (or staff) and had a very poor impact on making any improvements that people actually wanted (Weinstein, 2006), and the second approach, in which users took the lead, had the completely opposite effect.

How to manage service user involvement – some models

Wright et al. (2006, p13) recommend a whole systems approach to effective service user participation, of which many elements have also been explored in more detail in other chapters within this text. A whole systems approach incorporates four interacting elements (Wright et al., 2006). Firstly, the importance of culture where the ethos of an organisation demonstrates a commitment to participation; secondly that organisation's infrastructure, which needs to be able to facilitate any planning, development and resourcing of participation; thirdly, in direct practice, in which methods of working and the skills and knowledge of staff enable service users to become involved; and fourthly, the evidence that the organisation produces, through its monitoring and evaluation systems of any changes affected by participation and the ways in which these are reviewed. There are also different degrees of involvement such as those illustrated in the Stages Model discussed earlier (Arnstein, 1969; Pollitt, 2003).

At an individual level, people will be informed about the services available to them, then provide feedback about their care and service through service providers, commissioners or complaints procedures. Going on to the next stage at the individual level demonstrates the increasing influences of service users and the application of shared decisions about choices and options in care, leading to a situation where users take control over their own care and manage their own care arrangements perhaps by using direct payments or individualised budgeting. At a collective level, people can be informed about the type of services that are available and how well the services are performing, then provide feedback on their own experience; for example, through focus groups, other qualitative methods and surveys, to give a picture of what matters to service users and carers and what needs to be improved. At the next stage, service users can have influence through their representation on reference groups and decision-making bodies in relation to service reconfiguration or priority setting. Finally, users can be commissioners and providers of their own user-controlled services. There are still too few examples in social care of involvement moving beyond the level of consultation to one of control, indicating the need for a greater understanding of the complexity of user involvement, together with a practical knowledge of what needs to be put in place to support it.

Tokenism

As implied above, there is much more attention to service user involvement in 'safer' areas where the existence of focus groups on aspects of care and service user liaison groups remains at the periphery of decision-making. Social care is good at finding out what matters to services users, carers and the public, but less good at doing things about it (Community Care Needs Assessment Project, 2007). A significant shift is needed from feedback mode, where information is gathered about service users' experiences, to influence mode, where decision-making is shared with service users, carers and the public. Developing 'champions' of service user involvement who can lead at different levels within an organisation, without being isolated or overwhelmed by their participation in leading different operational and strategic tasks, might be one way forward. This area of work requires supportive networks in order to develop staff expertise, as facilitators, change-agents and finders of resources. Special attention will need to be given to developing participation within traditionally marginalised groups of users, who ironically are also more likely to be experiencing the poorest quality areas in the social care service system.

Professionals wishing to promote user involvement have frequently expressed concerns about the 'representativeness' of individual service users, sometimes suggesting that some of these may be 'too well', 'too articulate' or 'too vocal' to represent the views of users generally. This may be a subconscious method of resisting service user involvement or an inability to recognise service users as experts (Lindow, 1999). Achieving representative participation is not always easy and you will need to actively search for minority and marginalised groups in order to include their views. It is important to recognise that the more diverse a service user group, the more difficult it might be for any one person to represent them. For example, who can truly represent all disabled people?

CASE STUDY

In the City of Westminster, we found that black elders expressed views about personal care services that were very similar to the views of other people, focusing on reliability, honesty and trustworthiness. They were, however, more likely to emphasise gender concerns (black female users were more likely to prefer female care workers), request more appropriate food and voice concerns about discriminatory practices and racist comments. They appeared to have a low level of confidence in accessing systems to make complaints, and expressed interest in greater access to advocacy, and to information and advice about services. (Fieldwork study undertaken by the Nuffield Institute in 1997, cited in Martin and Henderson (2001, pp150–1))

For statutory services, including someone from the voluntary sector is not an adequate alternative to working directly with service users themselves. Users themselves are concerned about their own accountability (Community Care Needs Assessment Project, 2007). In order to maximise the potential for representativeness, you can support these individuals by providing funding and administrative support that promote the facilitation of more organised groups and an election process. Whilst some individuals may not necessarily be representative of other users, the legitimacy of their views rests in their personal experiences and how likely these are to have been shared by those in similar circumstances. Recognising and dealing with these dynamics is all part and parcel of the user involvement process. In conclusion, the roles in which people participate and their responsibilities are equally part of the process and will need to be discussed and clarified for all concerned (Community Care Needs Assessment Project, 2007).

Barriers to successful service user involvement

Despite increasing consultation and involvement, broader constraints remain that limit users' control over support services. A political emphasis on value for money, Best Value and restricting public expenditure can prioritise resource-driven services over needs-led or rights-led services where there are chronic problems of insufficient funding and service reductions. Beresford and Croft (2001) identify other constraints, such as the disablist and ageist nature of broader political and social structures and the low political priority attached to social work and welfare service users. They highlight the trend towards political centralisation and economic globalisation which has exerted pressure on public spending and employment conditions. Such structural barriers can also be expressed at a local level through the demonisation of particular service user groups, such as those with mental health issues or asylum seekers, and the longstanding culture of the service system, associated with restricted rights, inequality and stigmatisation for service users (Cowden and Singh, 2007). Top-down approaches to developing social care policy and making provision have meant that a particular range of interest groups, including politicians, managers, professionals, trade unions, planners and researchers has dominated the development and provision of services. Such provider-led services have been associated with a number of key failings and limitations. These include:

- a restriction on the rights of those people who use them;

- institutionalisation;

- an emphasis on social control;

- widespread abuse and neglect;

- shortcomings in standards;

- failure to ensure equal access and opportunities. (Beresford and Croft, 2001, p299)

The commissioning or contracting process is an area which has the potential to develop self-help approaches or community-led services. Local government in particular should be incentivised to engage constructively with user-led groups as service providers and their contribution to the strength of communities through capacity building and support for organisational development within the voluntary sector, which in turn can engage more service user involvement (Paxton and Pearce, 2005). Radical changes to what is measured under the comprehensive performance assessment used by central government to assess where local authorities are doing well may help to encourage this tactic. A recognition of niche skills and expertise, a proximity to service users, an ability to innovate and provide services flexibly by more secure and longer-term contracting with community-orientated and representative organisations as core providers of services, can all avoid perpetuating some of the problematic areas of practice within mainstream services (Bolton, 2003). Using independent, free-standing and small organisations to deliver services in this volatile environment inevitably increases the risk but this can be mitigated by a careful and rigorous approach to cost allocation and pricing which includes full cost recovery and an investment in building the business capacity of the recipient organisations (Paxton and Pearce, 2005).

CASE STUDY

Outcome-based commissioning

The development of outcome-based commissioning places an emphasis on the role of commissioners of services to commission services in outcome terms. For example, when looking at the high level outcomes of independence, wellbeing and choice (2005d) it can be difficult to define contracts in terms of a set of outcomes. One example is in the area of contracting for domiciliary care where the emphasis is often on the types, timings and costs of services being purchased. A more interactive dialogue between providers and commissioners is needed so that what providers do within a person's home contributes to the wider good of an individual and how this is articulated and evaluated. The other side of the coin may be the need to disinvest in services on the basis of outcomes they achieve and to determine whether a service value, given the amount of resources going in, is getting the yield of outcomes comparable with other services. This can help people to look at quality and outcome issues rather than just at cost and activity. Outcomes for individuals need to be very much expressed in people's own terms which are important to the choice agenda and control. Outcomes, for example around people becoming more independent, about well-being and health, will be different for different people. So enabling people to say in their own terms what the outcomes are that they are seeking to achieve from the service is critically important. This involves a huge culture-change involving a number of people, commissioners, contractors, service providers and of course managers and service users' input from the ground. (DoH, 2006a)

The above discussion questions how the outcomes stated in *Our health, our care, our say* (DoH, 2006a) can be translated into commissioning practices. This requires looking at the bigger picture, one where bodies such as the CSCI refocus performance indicators from being highly output-focused and at government level, via inspection regimes and work with statutory agencies. Being outcome-focused will need commissioning strategies at a local level to be able to separate output from outcomes, moving towards local area agreements, pooled budgets, and care groups where service users with social care and other professionals can explore the way resources can be used to invest in genuinely sought outcomes. This will inevitably involve other crucial players such as audit, finance, IT and lawyers, to develop more outcomes-based thinking (DoH, 2006a). All of this only serves to remind us of how complex it is to achieve outcomes-based approaches.

The importance of service user networks

Networking has been highlighted as an important benefit for service users to enable them to network with each other as individuals and in user-controlled organisations, both in terms of improving their quality of life and sustaining a more effective voice and presence to make a difference. Key obstacles that users identified in the way of individual networking included transport problems in rural areas, the fragility of user-controlled organisations and the effort of being involved (Beresford et al., 2006). Other barriers in the way of service user organisations networking include inadequate and insecure funding and resources.

Service user organisations generally do not have secure or reliable funding. Because of this, many service user organisations are liable to become led by funding issues rather than by their own concerns, priorities and principles, thus undermining their independence. The effects of inadequate and insecure funding can be divisive as service user-controlled organisations are placed under perverse pressure to compete with each other for the same resources. Smaller grassroots community-based organisations start off on an unequal footing by having to compete with big charitable organisations for funding. User-controlled organisations similarly may have a limited profile with big health, social care and educational commissioners of services.

Begum (2006) argues that there is a lack of local user-controlled organisations generally which disadvantages particular user groups, for example, young disabled people, people living with HIV/AIDS, disabled parents and black and minority ethnic communities, and this results in major gaps in service provision. By drawing attention to the inadequate provision for black and minority ethnic involvement in particular, Begum (2006) states that the mainstream service user movement cannot represent black and minority ethnic service users until race equality and anti-oppressive practice become integrated into everyone's everyday work (pviii). She notes that, whilst participation in the wider service user movement has gone from strength to strength, there has been a gradual decline of black and minority ethnic people with direct experience of requiring or using services, or being involved in shaping policy and practice to attain the outcomes that they want and need. The reasons are varied and complex, particularly since the history of black and minority ethnic people is rich in groundbreaking direct action and self-help. Begum warns against proxy participation through community 'leaders' and like Beresford et al. (2006) perceives that in practice, not all organisations which claim to be user-controlled are actually controlled by service users themselves. Black and minority voluntary sector organisations and black and minority ethnic professionals Begum recognises as having a role in advocating and representing service users' interests, but these are ultimately not immune to holding stereo-typical views of service users and their needs.

She concludes that there can be no substitute for the service participation of black and minority service users themselves and that service user movements in the UK are likely to be as racist as any other parts of society (2006, p15). It is important, therefore, for managers to be familiar with networks of users groups and organisations in the community and how these can be supported and leveraged to achieve more equality in relationships with them.

Involving young people and children

Children and young people can be involved in developing quality in social work and social care at a number of levels and there is already a lot of statutory guidance available to ensure that children are involved in all decisions relating to their care and education as far as possible (DfES, 2004; CSCI, 2005c). Innovative partnerships like the Lilac project described below and good practice examples of special con-sultation events or discussion groups to influence the design and provision of facilities and services are now increasing. Any action needs to reflect the age of the child or young person, their maturity and understanding, and the extent to which their parents and carers can also be involved. There is plenty of evidence to show that the effectiveness of services depends on listening and responding to children (Children and Young Persons' Unit, 2001) and that giving young people an active say in how policies and services are developed, provided, evaluated and improved can help those same policies and services to more genuinely meet their needs. Further, early engagement in public and community life is crucial to sustain-ing and building links with disadvantaged young people by giving them a role and the message that they really count and can contribute as a feature of citizenship (Children and Young Persons' Unit, 2001).

Children and young people need to be treated honestly, which means that their expectations are managed and that they are helped to understand the practical or legal boundaries of their involvement. Statutory services need to take a proactive approach in targeting those facing the greatest barriers to getting involved (for exam-ple, younger children, children and young people from minority ethnic backgrounds, those living in rural areas or disadvantaged neighbourhoods, children missing school, young people in the youth justice system, refugees, traveller children, disabled or other children with special needs, or children with special personal or family circum-stances) (Children and Young Persons' Unit, 2001). Where necessary, support and opportunities for training and development can be provided to children and young people so that they can contribute and participate effectively. Relevant information should be provided in good time and in appropriate formats, so that it is jargon-free, culturally appropriate and accessible.

CASE STUDY

Lilac (Lifelong Improvement for Looked-After Children) project is a groundbreaking pilot initiative in which young people who spent a large part of their own lives in care are training to become inspectors of LAs' care services. Lilac inspections will concentrate on how well LAs involve LAC in their own care, in the planning and evaluation of care services generally and on how effectively authorities handle complaints. The scheme is supported by CSCI and two LAs in West Sussex and York. The young people (in their 20s) themselves have developed the Lilac standards and will assess how strongly young people are involved in care, staff recruitment and in the choices given to LAC. The young people are being paid to train for the inspection work giving it professional status, and inspected services will receive a kite mark certifying their excellence at involving young people in improving services.
(*The Guardian*, 2007)

Practical issues for action

If your department or agency is to implement the participation and involvement of service users towards improving services, there are many practical issues to consider. (At the end of this chapter there is a list of publications and websites for specialist sources of advice.) Mapping current practice and expertise within your organisation as well as with key partners and agencies may show that there are already successful initiatives focused on involvement or that there is insufficient information or communication about what is already going on. Mapping helps to spread good practice and provides a baseline from which progress and improvement can be assessed, as well as highlighting any expertise available to assist your own service development. Being clear at the start about the objectives for any particular consultation or participation activity is essential. Honesty on all sides is needed about what is and is not likely to be influenced by service users and about how much decision-making can actually be shared with them; for example, where financial constraints or resource issues are involved. Power imbalances must be recognised by staff. There is often little time to make service users aware of all the factors involved and decisions made pragmatically by paid staff under pressure to meet deadlines may result in service users not feeling fairly consulted or satisfied.

At a minimal level, the use of *ad hoc* and routine suggestion schemes and opportunities for service users and carers through meetings in provider services can give feedback in the form of compliments and suggestions on current service provision. Formal surveys and questionnaires as we will see in the next chapter, can help to gauge opinion or explore users' more in-depth views about current services, gaps and particularly their subjective experiences. Any form of consultation implemented will need to utilise creative methods, particularly for those users who are not suited to traditional forms of communication or who have particular communication needs. Involving service users in direct consultation, or in leading participation activities as trainers, researchers, interviewers, recruitment panel members and mentors, is another way around this.

You could establish an advisory or decision-making body or ensure that other advisory or decision-making bodies have users in their membership on equal terms. Whichever approach is chosen, and often more than one is required, it is very important to tailor service user activities to the particular issues under consideration and outcomes being sought, as a 'one-size-fits-all' approach is not appropriate. If users are to participate on the same terms as professionals, they need the same opportunities to develop their skills to do so. Training needs identified by service users have included assertiveness and confidence-building courses run by user-trainers, equality training including legislation and policy, guidance on the decision-making structures for purchasers and providers of services and developing the necessary skills in negotiating and managing meetings. Training on any background issues must be done in an accessible way. Managers and staff can personally coach users on skills such as listening, how to present their views constructively or how to research information.

You should consider how service users and carers can receive recognition for their efforts. This might entail giving them a credit in a published document or speech for their input (Community Care Needs Assessment Project, 2007). As with staff, it is essential to exploring the links between users' progress in involvement activities with their personal learning and skills development. Activities around user involvement could be included on CVs, be given in a personal reference or can be accredited towards vocational or professional awards. The Commission for Social Care Inspection's Experts By Experience programme acknowledges that many people who use services are the true experts about their own situation and are closely involved by the CSCI to help the organisation develop its skills, knowledge and expertise in the inspection process (CSCI, 2007a).

Resourcing participation

User involvement, if properly implemented, can be financially expensive and time-consuming for organisations and service users alike. The principles and practice of reimbursing and paying service users for their involvement have been published in a document by the DoH (2006b) and this aims to provide some consistency of approach and to ensure that service users are treated fairly and appropriately according to their circumstances, so that they are able to make an informed choice about the arrangements concerning their involvement. The DoH guide was developed in consultation with relevant service user and patient organisations and health and social care organisations, and gives recognition to the issues around financial rewards and payment of expenses to service users in line with other contracted staff in social care. In order to meet costs and reimbursements, you will need to develop a budget and devise simple procedures for claiming expenses, so that those who are lacking in resources are not prevented from taking part because of financial barriers. Reimbursement should be easy to access; for example, through the provision of stamped addressed envelopes or methods of payment for people who do not hold bank accounts.

Staff development needs

The effective implementation of policies on service user participation often requires particular skills and experiences on the part of staff which should not be taken for granted within organisations delivering social care services. Staff need to be supported to think in new ways and be given the confidence and relevant development opportunities to try new approaches. Organisations with a good track record on these issues, including many led by service users and carers groups themselves, can help your own team develop realistic plans. They can assist you in thinking through when and how best to involve your service user group and can give specialist advice on what style of involvement is appropriate and the language or communication required. The involvement of an organisation in the voluntary sector, for example, can help to kick-start activities and then offer ongoing support. In Chapter 3 we talked about dispersed and situational leadership and the potential for identifying someone from your service area or team with sufficient influence and the skills and interest to champion this area of work. As we discussed earlier, users are not a homogeneous group and there is no single way to involve them. This means considering methods that incorporate advocacy, translators, interpreters and mixed media such as new technologies. Particularly challenging to involve are those members of the community who have previous adverse experiences of services. Utilising the support of groups that already have relationships with those members can be helpful.

As a starting point, whatever level of participation you are promoting and whatever phase you are in, you should always anticipate and be ready to deal with difficulties; for example, where people do not read your leaflets or attend meetings. Similarly, different interest groups may have conflicting aims, colleagues may fail to deliver and you may end up as the scapegoat for everyone's difficulties (Kotecha et al., 2007)! Reducing the potential for failure can be met by good planning around access arrangements, the timing and frequency of meetings, and the use of a variety of contact-means including electronic. The venue and its associations for any meetings are important, as is available, easy and low cost transport which may need to be arranged or accompanied. Arrangements for carers are also essential. Confidentiality needs to be clarified, perhaps by developing and agreeing a written protocol that is understood and accepted by everyone. An agreement and clarity about how the information and views that users share with those working with them will be used should be drawn up. This is particularly useful if there is a significant turnover of staff, where users and staff have previously become familiar with each other and both groups have to start all over again. Finally, in order to avoid consultation fatigue, Carr (2004) talks about the importance of following up and giving feedback from any involvement activity within an appropriate timescale. Feedback to users following their participation needs to make clear what is intended in the short-, medium- and long-term and should explain why particular suggestions or priorities could not be taken forward. Participation activities should be honestly evaluated; not all approaches will be successful and mistakes will be made, but it is important that lessons are learned, shared and built upon.

Social care and social work professionals all have an important role to play in promoting user participation. Whilst some circumstance can limit participation in decision-making, for example because of legal and professional obligations such as childcare proceedings, a clarity that recognises service users as citizens can promote social inclusion. Begum (2006, p19) tells us that there is much to be learnt from other social movements about how people who are not members of a particular group (such as non-disabled people, white people and heterosexuals) can be allies and open doors that may not otherwise be accessible. The assumption that empowerment and participation require professionals to take a back seat is short-sighted and naïve, because there are times when the support and power of professionals are really necessary (Begum, 2006). Likewise, caution needs to be exercised to avoid some of the pitfalls of participation work, for example, the formal meetings and paperwork that may not actually be appropriate or relevant to the users with whom one is working and which can disadvantage them (Trivedi, 2002).

Planning service user participation in quality improvements

If you are involving service users in quality improvements, set priorities and begin in a small way. Make sure that user participation in particular policy and service areas is proportional to the relevance of the issues to users themselves. Participation might begin in some priority areas and be expanded across other departmental areas once experience and capacity have been built up. Putting these into a local and departmental policy might include the following which have been recommended by Community Care Needs Assessment Project, 2007; Kotecho et al., 2007;

- Strategies for implementing the core principles.

- Your priorities for action and timescales for implementing the strategies.

- How you will make a visible commitment to participation in accordance with the principles.

- An outline of specific events or initiatives envisaged and structures for involvement put in place at a local level.

- How capacity within your department is being developed and supported.

- Plans for evaluating participation activities.

- Monitoring and reporting arrangements about progress with a view to producing an annual report of participation activities in your department and making sure that these do not duplicate or confuse action going on in other agencies or organisations.

- Using the above to commission further work to identify, assess and disseminate the positive benefits of participation policies and services from the involvement of users and carers. This may include publishing the effective approaches and best practice for giving service users and carers real choices over some of the important issues that your organisation and others like it are tackling in their work.

Customer complaints and representation procedures

Complaints is an area of quality control that has emerged since the 1989 NHS and community care reforms, with the development of procedures and systems to enable users to make direct representations about many aspects of care and its quality. There are, however, several gaps in the linkages between complaints and modern ideas about systematic quality improvement (Bell and Osborne, 2005). The development of national and local charters and standards in particular has placed an emphasis on improving quality by using complaints to create change in both health and social care services. Regardless of this, it must be recognised that complaints focus on quality at the point of weakness or failure, rather than at the strategic level.

Complaints, however, do provide a useful source in evaluating aspects of service quality and therefore have a role as part of the overall effort to achieve effective quality management and clinical governance. There are ways in which they can be systematically employed to create widespread service improvement. These might include reflecting in your teams or services on recurring issues in a problem-solving way, using service users themselves to assist in investigating complaints and the support of service user advocates at an early stage in the complaint to help those likely to complain or pursue a complaint (Berman Brown and Bell, 1998). Bell and Osborne (2005) undertook a content analysis of literature in health care around complaints and found that there was a greater emphasis on professional and managerial rather than service user views of quality. Rebalancing these perspectives in the literature can help to expand our knowledge about the impact of complaining at both the theoretical and empirical levels.

Whilst complaints *per se* are an important indicator of quality, however, a lack of complaints does not necessarily indicate the presence of quality. Services users are themselves often reluctant to complain for a number of reasons. Complaints are based on a paradigm of defects rather than on strategic quality, reflecting the different approaches to quality assurance discussed in Chapter 2. There is also significant evidence that patterns of complaining in certain areas have not necessarily effected change (Simon, 1995).

Finally, it has been argued that current mechanisms for dealing with complaints from vulnerable people remain procedurally- rather than person-driven, and may represent a hidden iceberg of lost complaints in services delivered to this group. A review of any complaints procedures in your team will need to consider whether there are any gaps between complaints and safeguarding policies and the ability of complainants to fulfil the requirements of such policies. For vulnerable adults, the Mental Incapacity Act 2006 has to some extent filled one of the gaps in relation to the potential of advocacy and opportunities to develop advocacy services. However, in your own service, giving attention to the support offered by staff to help users and carers effectively pursue complaints where appropriate, cannot be underestimated.

Involving mental health service users in quality assurance

We are going to conclude this chapter by looking at a specific best practice example of involving service users in a quality assurance initiative. It remains the norm for managers and researchers to design questionnaires, interviews and inventories around quality assurance that reflect their own interests and concerns. These may not, however, reflect the priorities of service users.

User-focused monitoring has been developed at the Sainsbury Centre for Mental Health since 1996, starting from the premise that if the evaluation of services was to genuinely reflect the concerns and views of the people who use them rather than those of providers, then users should lead the process at every stage. This starts with composing the questions asked, through to the collection, analysis and interpretation of data, to the final reporting of the results and the development of recommendations for change (Kotecha et al., 2007).

CASE STUDY

Weinstein (2006) compared two quality assurance reviews in a voluntary sector organisation centre for mental health for a particular ethnic group. The first was a professional-led process and the second a user-led process. Her comparison illuminated how different the agenda of the service users was compared with the agenda of staff when users were asked to identify their priorities. The users did not prioritise care plans, reviews or even aspects of key working (which were the main areas reviewed in the professional-led process two years previously). The concerns of service users were mostly about their own quality of life as human beings and as members of a community; they wanted to go on holiday like other people and they hated feeling lonely and isolated when the service was closed on a bank holiday. Whilst service users appreciated having a structure to their day, the most important aspect of the Centre from their perspective was that it provided a safe haven where they felt comfortable and accepted among their own community.

Addressing some of these issues began a process of further development of day services that was more outward-looking and enabled users to participate more actively in the life of the community. The user-led project played a part in the evolution of QA within the organisation, helping it to develop from:

- *focusing on an inspection event to focusing on an QA process;*

- *the customer being a 'vague concept' to the customer being a 'specific person or group with specific needs';*

- *quality being the responsibility of the quality department to quality being the responsibility of every employee. (Weinstein, 2006)*

Details about the different approaches taken at each level in this case study are demonstrated in Table 4.1 on p80. As an example of good practice, by repeating a process like this at regular intervals, a team or service can progressively implement user-focused practice and service developments, and can evaluate the impact of these on user experience in a continuing cycle of improvement (Kotecha et al., 2007).

Table 4.1 A comparison between two QA reviews in a mental health day centre in the voluntary sector

Quality assurance process	First review	Second review
Planning process	Discussion between Director of service and Director of QA unit	Steering group composed of service users, day centre staff, volunteers, QA team members and external service user consultant
QA process	One day event	Six month process
Purpose of the questionnaire Survey	Designed directly to identify how far service standards were being met	Designed to explore the priorities identified by service users themselves
Wording in the questionnaire	Drafted by the QA unit	Drafted by the QA steering group and revised after pilot with eight service users
How the questionnaire was distributed	Distributed by day centre staff to users who came into the centre during a two week period	Posted to the home address of each service user
Return of the questionnaire	Questionnaires returned to the day centre	Questionnaires returned in sealed SAE envelopes directly to the QA unit
Consultation with staff	Two members of staff interviewed on the day of the QA review	Manager and staff represented on steering group and full consultation of the staff team on the draft questionnaire and involved throughout the process
Response rate	28 per cent	73 per cent
Report	Analysed and written by QA unit with judgements and recommendations	Analysed and written by QA unit setting out the user responses and no judgements or recommendations
Feedback of findings	Presented to Director of service and Board of Trustees with recommendations	Presented to service users and staff for them to decide on a plan of action
Outcome	Staff indifference and user cynicism – no system for monitoring implementation of recommendations.	Service users and staff agreed an action plan and monitoring process

(Source: Weinstein, 2006) *Reprinted with kind permission of Blackwell Publishing.*

C H A P T E R   S U M M A R Y

The attainment of independence and autonomy in an outcome-based approach to providing quality services has implications for services and structures that typically go beyond the remit of health or social care services. These take into account issues around social inclusion, the nature of the built environment and wider citizen social and economic participation. From the point of view of service users, the way in which organisations respond to their needs, the ease of access to services and the degree to which these are flexible and meet their needs and preferences are always likely to be important aspects of quality. The participation and involvement of service users in the design, delivery and evaluation of services provide an important way of assessing these aspects. Assessing the quality of the process can be done comprehensively on a wider scale using some of the suggestions given above, or on a day-to-day basis regarding the ways in which we ask service users what they think and feel about our interactions with them. Performance measurement or quality indicators which seem plausible to us should be tested before being used, to see if they really are related to the outcomes that matter most to service users themselves. This is illustrated in the example of the user-led quality assurance review in the mental health day centre.

Whatever the nature of service provision in years to come, the need for services to be evaluated from the standpoint of people who use them has never been greater. This is a political issue where a huge chasm remains between the political imperatives of managing risk and the imperatives of creating services that are enabling and provide real support and safety (Kotecha et al., 2007). Establishing and sustaining user participation and involvement in your service may be at an early stage or already well advanced. Whatever the situation, meaningful service user involvement takes time, energy and commitment and cannot be reduced to a management imperative. Cowden and Singh (2007) leave us with some final words on this issue:

> *rather than allowing this to become another item for managers to tick off, front-line staff should reclaim the agenda of critical practice and argue for this not just as a vehicle for social inclusion, but most critically, in the longer term, as a means by which new insights into power and powerlessness can be gained and new emancipatory policies constructed. (p 21)*

FURTHER READING

Turner, M and Beresford, P (2005) *Contributing on equal terms: service user involvement and the benefits system.* Bristol: Policy Press.
Published by SCIE with Shaping Our Lives, this report draws on relevant literature and has involved a wide range of service users and other stakeholders in discussions about the issues involved in payment for participation. It explores in detail the range of difficulties arising for people using services and the organisations seeking their involvement, and makes recommendations for improving policy and practice in the field.

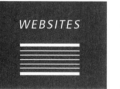

WEBSITES

National Black Youth Forum: infodesk@nationalblackyouthforum.org.uk
A children- and young person-led organisation that exists to protect and promote the rights of children and young people of Asian, African and Caribbean heritage in the UK. The organisation aims to promote good race relations between these groups and wider society by combating discrimination in all its manifestations. The Forum is able to offer departments the resource of young people as advisers or speakers and is also happy to offer telephone support and advice to departments.

A National Voice: office@anv.u-net.com
Run by and for young people who are or have been in care, they are a mixed group from all over England. The organisation aims to get rid of the poor image of young people in care, to stop mistreatment of young people in care, and to have an effect on government decisions about the care system. A National Voice can provide advice on the phone, information about good practice,

signposting to other sources of information and access to groups of children and young people for training and consultation.

Common Purpose: Just Do Something: www.justdosomething.net
Aims to help people in leadership and decision-making positions to be more effective in their own organisations and community in citizen participation and has a 'How To' resource.

Better government for older people: www.bettergovernmentforolderpeople.gov.uk
Describes successful initiatives to engage older people and has a formal management structure with a majority of older people as an example of citizen involvement at a strategic level.

Central England People First: www.peoplefirst.org.uk
Run and controlled by people with learning difficulties and providing accessible information and advocacy.

National Centre for Independent Living: www.ncil.org.uk
Provides information, training, expertise and policy development on all aspects of independent living.

Chapter 5

Using evidence and evaluation to improve services

ACHIEVING POST-QUALIFYING SOCIAL WORK AWARDS

If you are a registered social worker, this chapter will assist you to evidence post-registration training and learning. It relates to the national post-qualifying framework for social work education and training, in particular the national criteria at the higher specialist/advanced level.
* *ix Support, mentor, supervise or manage others, exercising practice, research, management or educational leadership to enable them to identify and explore issues and improve their own practice.*

And it will also help you develop to the leadership and management standards in social care.
* *C1 Encourage innovation in your team – encouraging people to improve current services and ways of doing things by developing a climate where people feel able to think creatively about practice, systems and processes.*
* *C2 Encourage innovation in your area of responsibility – to support the identification and practical implementation of ideas, primarily from people in your area of responsibility, for improving existing services and developing new services.*

Introduction

Improving services requires the engagement of the social care workforce in identifying priorities for integrating knowledge with existing and future practice. All staff need to be able to construct a reliable basis of testing the day-to-day feasibility of interventions and their effectiveness. Current debates about performance management and the introduction of quality improvement systems provide a unique opportunity to question how far the evaluation of the effectiveness of social care supplies objective, impartial evidence for decision-making and public accountability, and generates knowledge about social policy, social problems and how best to solve them (Shaw, 2004). In order to engage in these debates we need to be clear about what infrastructure exists for creating and disseminating knowledge, the different sources of evidence in social care and to understand our relationship with these. We will also want to consider how far evidence, knowledge or research provides us with a deliverable platform to take forward the integrated care agenda where, increasingly, agreement for common policies and practices is required in very diverse professional cultures.

Webb (2006) talks about the social and cultural embeddedness of important knowledge constructs in social work and how these set the parameters for front-line practice. Practice can vary widely depending on situational factors and adherence to particular models of practice. It is also affected by the priorities given to certain policies, and resources and by the influence of managers. In this respect, the boundaries of social work knowledge are always to some degree unstable because of its shifting relationship between its authoritative sources, reference points and other professional contexts across time (Webb, 2006). All these point to a need for a more critical evaluation of which areas of research and theory get invoked in practice. We also need to evaluate the research and theory we use and its relationship with our knowledge about service users and their difficulties, as discussed in the previous chapter. Managers and leaders of quality improvements will of course need to take an active role in this respect.

This chapter will begin by looking at the development of the evidence-based practice debate in social work and how this has been defined and characterised. We will review the limitations of evidence-based or evidence-informed practice and the problems it raises as set out by some commentators who have questioned its usefulness and application. We will interrogate how practitioners and managers use knowledge and acknowledge the different types of knowledge-making process inherent in practice (Taylor and White, 2006). Commitments to certain forms of knowledge can bring with them epistemological assumptions or constraints on the range of action and interventions subsequently chosen. These are important issues in the context of evidence-based practice and management in social care. Many management techniques selected for enhancing effectiveness, efficiency and productivity reflect a set of beliefs or doctrines about how evidence-based practice should be taken forward. This chapter is particularly concerned with highlighting the importance of practice wisdom and the lived experiences of service users/carers in judging the accuracy and quality of different types of knowledge and evaluation in social care. The latter will follow up on our discussions from the previous chapter on service user participation. This chapter will conclude with some practical pointers for how you might go about undertaking your own evaluation or in-house research studies which build on knowledge and the evidence required for quality improvement and judging performance.

Evidence-based practice, definitions and characteristics

One of the preoccupations of the modernisation agenda in social care has been to generate and disseminate evidence of sufficient quality and quantity to underpin national policy-making and to develop practice knowledge. This has grown in parallel with relevant and appropriate research activity to move this agenda forward and to encourage a more applied approach to generating knowledge using systematic reviews (Macdonald, 2003). Evidence-based social care is defined as *the conscientious, explicit and judicious use of current best evidence in making decisions regarding the welfare of those in need* (Sheldon and Chilvers, 2000, p5, based on Sackett et al., 1996, p71). Marsh et al. (2005, p3) try to capture the exact role of *evidence* in the knowledge base for social care by citing the following formula:

Knowledge = evidence + practice wisdom + service user and carer experiences and wishes

This formula is valuable because it does not imply any hierarchy within the three components of knowledge except that they can vary in importance depending on the question under consideration. Marsh et al. (2005) clarify that the meaning of *evidence* in this construction as being derived from that which is generated by research findings and its interpretation. They propose that any research-based evidence must be relevant and applicable to practice concerns in a way that engages with the interests of practitioners, users and carers and which includes their experiences in providing and receiving services (p3).

The relationship between social work practice and its knowledge has been the subject of a long ongoing debate which we were made aware of in Chapter 1 when looking at the historical development of performance management. Despite the clear location of social work training within higher education, this debate has remained inconclusive and is characterised by the existence of two cultures in social work; one which emphasises prescriptions and learning from direct practice and which would appear to have considerable intuitive appeal, and the other coming from a more academic environment which places a high value on theory, validity and evidence in the scientific tradition (Sheppard et al., 2000). Since the modernisation of social care from the 1990s, growing interest in the skills mix and the blurring of professional boundaries have together served to prolong the scepticism about the importance and use of knowledge in practice. This is combined with concerns about whether sufficiently sophisticated methodologies have been able to provide the necessary skills available to generate knowledge and to meet the specific needs of social care agencies and their users (Sheppard et al., 2000). This concern has certainly been taken up in the recent revision of post-qualifying awards in social work, particularly in the higher specialist and advanced levels where you are required to demonstrate an *enhanced level of competence in applied professional research and work effectively and creatively as a researcher in an area of risk, conflict, uncertainty or where there are complex challenges and a need to make a balanced judgement* (Requirement vi, GSCC, 2005).

Other criticisms of evidence-based practice highlight the positivistic standpoint of its proponents. The process of knowledge application in this paradigm is seen as unproblematic and values a clear hierarchy of methods used to generate evidence about social care. Whilst this has been seen as an attempt to provide some certainty in the face of the many complexities facing social care service delivery, the claim that policy and practice should be evidence-based is, according to Glasby and Beresford (2006), a *statement of a dilemma and not as a complete blueprint for the way forward* (p 269). For example, the more rigorous the research design, the more transparent and applicable the findings are considered to be. Glasby and Beresford, however, question what constitutes valid evidence and especially who decides what types of evidence should be treated as more legitimate than others (2006, p269).

The need to summarise the extent of our current knowledge on particular topics has been supported through a number of government-sponsored mechanisms. For example, the Policy Research Programme (PRP) is a national programme of research dedicated to providing an evidence-base for policy-making in the Department of Health (DoH, 2007). This programme works alongside other national research programmes and consults when necessary with policy research programmes in other government departments and a wide variety of stakeholders. This builds further on the introduction of evidence-based frameworks for various health and social care services and the appearance of national bodies which disseminate research and evidence, such as the National Institute for Clinical Effectiveness and the Social Care Institute for Excellence. Statistical surveys at national and local levels can also provide important information about trends, along with findings from inspection and audits on service performance. Systematic reviews and randomised controlled trials are seen as the gold standard of social care research, both of which use approaches associated traditionally with science and health care research and are perceived as implementing the most objective methods.

However, some experimental designs which privilege a scientific and quantifiable approach are clearly not the most appropriate method where practice presents us with considerable and unquantifiable challenges. Randomised control trials might be the most appropriate approach in evaluative research or in outcome studies, where the outcome or output of an intervention can be clearly specified in advance; for example, where you are assessing the types and quantities of service provided such as domiciliary care versus direct payments offered.

Yet exploratory research which seeks to capture qualitative data or expert opinion can also be valuable as an emancipatory means of capturing or acquiring knowledge. These are equally important to the discipline of social work, where practice is a complex, uncertain and ambiguous activity which involves an ethical base and legal accountability. It is extremely difficult to capture data about complex assessments and decision-making encompassing relative risks, safety, harm and protection and the interventions chosen (Lishman, 2000). In summary then, tensions between these different methods when we are talking about evidence or knowledge reflect the complex context in which social work practice can be measured or evaluated, but also render problematic any simple definitions of the nature of evidence-based practice.

Why do we need knowledge based on evidence in social work?

Despite reservations, and before exploring the different sources of knowledge in social work and social care further, it is useful to rehearse the main arguments initially outlined in Chapter 1 for why we need such knowledge and what evidence from research contributes to social care. If you recall, these were succinctly summarised by Marsh et al. (2005, pp3–4) as follows.

- Decisions taken by social care professionals have a major impact on the *immediate* life chances of service users and carers and well-informed practitioners are vital to ensuring best quality immediate outcomes for highly disadvantaged people.

- The impact over time of decisions on *the longer-term life chances* of service users and carers will have substantial implications for their quality of life and, therefore, best informed practice is the right of those people whose long-term outcome depends in part on social care decisions.

- Good evidence challenges fundamental assumptions about social care which may bring substantial advantages to service users and carers. Some research, such as that done in the area of direct payments and the effectiveness of family group conferences, has revolutionised the concept of expertise by demonstrating the potential of service users' control of their own lives, giving rise to major and sometimes controversial shifts in policy-making and resource provision.

- In substantial areas of social care where strong powers or compulsion are exercised, for example by courts, providing the best evidence helps to put in place safeguards in decision-making.

- An informed public can engage better with relevant debates about services and will need access to the best evidence to do so.

- Informed service user and carer communities and individuals are able to use evidence to facilitate direct involvement in services and engagement with their development.

There are also claims that go beyond the rational use of evidence outlined above which entail the *conscientious, judicious and explicit* terms used in the definition of evidence-based practice presented earlier (Sackett, 1997, p71). These terms suggest that there is also a moral duty. It acknowledges the implicit sound judgement of professionals which in turn expresses a mark of their practical wisdom and discretion. The term 'explicit' claims transparency and openness where nothing is left implied. However, we know that professional judgement also involves accountability and is based on moral reasoning (Shaw, 2004).

Different types of knowledge used in social care

In organisational terms, knowledge is an important strategic asset (Clegg et al., 2005) and there has been increasing interest in the concept of knowledge management as a tool for increasing effectiveness and competitiveness based on the experiences of the industry and business sector. Social care is an area rich with knowledge. Knowledge management describes the process by which knowledge is created, stored, distributed and applied to decision-making. This 'theory' first became prominent when change management was linked with management learning by Senge (1990). In relation to the care sector, Pawson et al. (2003) have explored and reviewed the types and quality of social care knowledge available and they have developed a useful classification system. This is based on two aspects: firstly, by examining the process through which knowledge is created (for example through audit, review, survey, trial or evaluation) and secondly, by examining the vehicle through which knowledge is disseminated (for example academic literature, education and training, policy and procedures at work), as well as through less formal measures.

This approach, like others already referred to in this chapter so far, dismisses any hierarchy in knowledge production, but points to the potential for making quality judgements about a particular piece of evidence from each source. There are five source domains offered by Pawson et al. (2003), the first of which is *organisational knowledge* which provides a comprehensive accountability framework mostly via governance and regulatory activities. There are also a number of external bodies which promote and govern national standards and which lay down what is minimally acceptable. It is often taken for granted that these standards are easily or actually implemented and evaluated and particularly because of the complex national and local apparatus of training, inspection, audit and inquiry that appear to do this. However, highly performing organisations tend to consult a wider range of stake-holders and are more aspirational in setting standards which enable them in addition to appraise and interact with their own local knowledge base (Clegg et al., 2005). Organisations grappling with more difficult issues, such as outcomes of certain interventions or those that are dynamic in developing risk management or risk aversion standards, are more likely to learn and develop their knowledge base.

The second domain concerns *practitioners' knowledge* which will be explored further in Chapter 6. This refers to the idea of reflective practice which lies at the heart of practitioners' knowledge and is acquired through the distillation of collective wisdom at many points, such as through education and training, supervision and consultation, team working as well as personal approaches where practitioners judge their efforts in terms of emotional rewards, peer approval, service user feedback and 'gut reaction'. Practitioners' knowledge tends to be personal and context specific and therefore difficult to surface, articulate and aggregate. At the same time, practitioners' knowledge can operate through a highly systematic analytical and critical process concentrating on common issues pertinent to their direct work with service users.

The third domain follows on from the previous chapter, that of *users and carers*, where the development of user-led and emancipatory research based on the social model has contributed to a knowledge base which increases users' choice and control over their own lives and involves them in all decisions about the delivery of services.

The fourth domain is *research knowledge* as outlined above in the previous section and is among the most palpable source of social care knowledge derived from empirical inquiries which are based on predetermined research strategies. The reports, evaluations, assessments and measures from these form the most orthodox items in any evidence base. Debates about transparency, accuracy, purposivity and propriety, as well as issues about ethics and quality, need to be further developed in social care research (Pawson et al., 2003). We will look later on at how managers can encourage critical appraisal of research-based evidence so that practitioners can judge its quality and relevance and ensure that this is an essential skill and competency for continuing professional development in social care.

Finally, *policy and community knowledge* sets social care in its wider policy context by providing knowledge about what social care does and how it might fit into its complex political, social and economic environment. Structural models to understand social problems and issues and vital knowledge about the organisation and implementation of services are derived from the broader policy community. The key contributors to policy community knowledge includes central, regional and local government and its agencies and the members of think tanks, lobby groups, policy and research staff in political parties and scholars of public policy (Pawson et al., 2003).

As you can see, knowledge itself is increasingly seen as a product, something tangible such as a set of information or that which can be written down and subsequently

accessed and used in practice. This is a particular assumption underlying the proponents of evidence-based practice. Alongside this notion, knowledge is also seen as a
process which draws on the cognitive processes by which understanding is created
and in particular processes associated with hypothesis testing. This is a particular ideal
underpinning reflective learning and critically reflective practice. Both types of knowledge are complementary because process knowledge can inform the ways in which
formal product knowledge can be related to practice alongside lessons from other life
and practice experiences. Sheppard (1995) claims that we do not as yet have process
knowledge for social work, implying the need for more empirical work through which
process knowledge can be developed and incorporated into rigorous cognitive processes which can be taught for social work practice.

Formal and informal knowledge

So far, we have generally been talking about explicit, theoretically-based knowledge,
albeit, from a range of sources which is not difficult to conceptualise and is more
easily stored and accessible (Polanyi, 1983). In the last decade however, management
theorists have noted that tacit knowledge, which is that derived from practice and
experience, contributes significantly to innovation processes. Tacit knowledge is context specific and consists of personal beliefs, values and perspectives that individuals
take for granted in their day-to-day practice. It is important for managers and practitioners to know how to organise and manage tacit knowledge and how to transform
elements from it into explicit organisational knowledge. However, most knowledge
management approaches consist only of storing explicit knowledge.

Commentators from the social constructionist school (Lave and Wenger, 2002) have
highlighted the important interactive social process of creating and sharing knowledge. A 'community of practice' is their term for how people learn naturally in their
work communities and this emphasises practice over theory and social learning over
individual learning, and is put forward as a good environment for the development of
evidence-based practice. Within any 'community', members will have different interests, will make diverse contributions to the activities that go on and will hold various
viewpoints. Participation in learning about practice can take place at multiple levels
and is a shared responsibility by those within it, whether they are in virtual or co-
located groups. A community of practice may not necessarily imply co-presence, a
well defined and identifiable group, or a socially visible boundary, which makes it
particularly attractive within multi-disciplinary care environments. It does, however,
imply participation in a system about which participants share a common understanding about what they are doing, a common knowledge base and what this means for
the quality of the service as a whole. The developmental cycles of that community
provide access to a wide range of information, resources and opportunities for service
improvement through participation. Managers can nurture these cycles by using
opportunities for developing quality circles, by encouraging research and evaluation
as integral activities, by actively collaborating with people producing research, and by
making time available for practitioners to share their knowledge (Hafford-Letchfield et
al., 2007).

Sandars (2004) talks more about the knowledge management *process* which enables organisations to manage both tacit and explicit knowledge. The first step is where one creates explicit new knowledge from research and this is tapped into through the day-to-day experiences of practitioners who internalise this explicit knowledge and convert it into tacit knowledge – the so-called 'evidence base'. Within any organisation, explicit knowledge can be stored in a variety of formats, the most common being IT- or library-based. However, tacit knowledge is more difficult to articulate and store as it is embodied within the notion of managers', practitioners' and service users' 'expertise'. Staff can possibly access these via techniques of consultation, supervision or coaching or by the observation of another's practice which we commonly recognise as work-based learning. Sandars (2004) is particularly concerned with how knowledge is utilised for problem-solving and decision-making. The provision of knowledge at the right point and its translation into practice are essential tasks of knowledge management and communities of practice described above can prove a good vehicle here.

Professional knowledge

The potential for encouraging reflective practice as a tool for quality improvement is enormous and refers to the process where practitioners build up exemplary themes through their case experiences – which, in subsequent scenarios, they can draw on and compare and thus create new meanings to inform their subsequent actions (Schon, 1991). Whilst this is not an explicit experimental process, practitioners will question their situation and develop a hypothesis. Practioners then actively seek confirmatory evidence through their involvement to influence the situation so that the hypothesis is confirmed. According to Sheppard et al. (2000), this is essential to their reframing of the situation. This way of working in practice has led to a study of expertise through which researchers have sought to discover the key elements of 'expert practice' (Benner, 2001).The practice of reflection relies on the importance of intuition and practice wisdom in the reasoning process of experts, who may be unable to articulate with any clarity their cognitive processes in professional decision-making, but are nevertheless able to engage in forward reasoning. Boud and Walker (2002) remind us that the very nature of reflective activities is such that they may lead to serious questioning and critical thinking whereby a learner challenges the assumptions of managers or the practice context in which they are operating. A recognition of affective dimensions of learning and practice means that this can thrive only in a climate in which the expression of feelings in accepted and legitimate, for example within supervision and team communication.

Communicating knowledge in practice

Social workers, like all professionals, claim their professional status on the basis of their practice being rooted in a sound knowledge base, ethical standards and codes of practice as well as their being able to communicate the basis of their decision-making and practice to others (Osmond and O'Connor, 2004). The capacity of social work professionals to articulate their practice knowledge is not only essential for the issue of accountability, but also in order to enhance the likelihood of providing quality in service delivery.

Osmond and O'Connor (2004) undertook an empirical study into how social work practitioners actually express and explain what they know. This was done with a view to ascertaining whether or not formalised education and research are serving the needs of practice. They found that knowledge expressed by practitioners was not always formal or labelled, but was often given via examples, stories and metaphors, as well as understandings that resembled existing theoretical knowledge or that which had been reformulated and synthesised in practice. Metaphors, for example, can assist in uplifting tacit understanding (p684).

Their study specifically brought to the fore two main issues for consideration: firstly, that knowledge can be implied or inferred in practice language, and secondly, that practitioners can have difficulty in articulating and naming the basis of their work. They recommended that the issue of competent and clear practice articulation is a topic to which the profession should give serious attention. Educative and supervisory attention was considered important for future practice behaviour by strengthening practitioners' capacity to articulate what they know. This could involve training practitioners or students in critical reflective techniques, knowledge articulation and systematic approaches to practice.

The inability of practitioners in their view, to explicitly articulate the basis of practice behaviour places social workers at a considerable disadvantage in a competitive labour market. Osmond and O'Connor recommended that practice knowledge will benefit from reflective analysis which allows underlying and tacit assumptions to surface. This could lead to tacit knowledge being extended or exposed for critique or empirical testing. Finally, in an acknowledgement of the state-sponsored activities social work carries out, the issue of knowledge for accountability is crucial and has a strong connection with outcomes for service users.

Performance management information – another source of knowledge?

So far, we have been talking about sources of knowledge in social care and how much these are tangible and able to be translated into practice, particularly in the case of research-based knowledge. Performance management systems imply in some way that knowledge and its application are integrated into service delivery and are geared up to assess any outcome from these. The introduction of performance management systems and improvements in information technology has given rise to a plethora of returns of detailed information on interventions and outputs in care services which provides an enormous source of 'knowledge' by which we can measure aspects of quality or performance. This is what is commonly known as 'audit' activity and is usually presented in the form of a series of tables accompanied by bulletins to interpret trends or issues. Many big organisations employ information officers with the technical and analytical skills to explore the organisations' own data which, in the past, used to be almost exclusively collected and interpreted by researchers (Ward, 2004, p14). Whoever collects and analyses this type of information within an organisation, it is certainly good practice to disseminate any findings for the purposes of improving care services and to help staff and team's practice development.

Paxton et al. (2006) compare some activities of research and audit which they say are similar in several respects. These attempt to answer specific questions through collecting and analysing data, although research is mainly concerned with discovering the right thing to do whereas audit is concerned with ensuring that it is done right (Smith, 1992). Clarifying the difference helps to identify the various mechanisms and processes needed to ensure quality and to manage risk in both research and audit (Paxton et al., 2006). The Department of Health's research governance standards recognise that associated with acquiring new knowledge is the likelihood of bringing more risks (DoH, 2005c). Audit, on the other hand, is not subject to the same stringent external requirements and is more likely to be concerned with assessing current projects against existing good practice standards. Paxton et al. (20006) still highlight the ethical imperative to monitor and regulate audit and other related activities (such as evaluation, as we will see below). They note that the closeness of the scrutiny and the assessment standards will be in proportion to the likely lower risk.

Audit is a very important activity for quality assurance and assessing performance. If it is undertaken cyclically, it can assess current services against standards set and take steps to bring practice in line with such standards, review these again, and so on. The primary purpose of audit is to improve the quality of a service or intervention by promoting adherence to standards. Good practice and innovative work on audit, as with research, should be disseminated as the main use of audit data. The reason for carrying out an audit is to improve or maintain practice in line with standards set. As someone who may have audit activity going on in your service area, you will probably want to develop manageable systems to follow up improvement projects and to collect and share information on their outcomes – the impact could be of great value in spreading service improvement.

A possible link or step between audit and research is evaluation. Evaluation can be defined as the task of working out whether a course of action is effective (Axford et al., 2005), perhaps using audit information. Alternatively it can be done for research purposes and to inform development work aimed at improving interventions. Axford et al. (2005) define four primary requirements of effective evaluation: firstly, to focus on a specific group of service users who might benefit from the intervention being evaluated, and secondly, to decide what should be done to help a user or group of users i.e. the intervention. Thirdly, to find out whether the intervention was delivered as intended, and fourthly, to evaluate whether or not that course of action achieved its stated objectives. The remainder of this chapter is going to look at evaluation as a method that you can use to plan for improving services.

Using evaluation techniques to identify and plan for service improvements

Evaluation is part and parcel of everyday professional activity. If you are a manager or senior practitioner, you are likely to be at the interface between the many procedures and operations involved in making judgements about the value of alternative courses of action within a wide organisational context. You might be asked to evaluate something that has gone wrong; for example, following a complaint or critical incident.

Evaluation is a deliberate and explicit management activity that builds on the processes of performance management. As outlined above, evaluation assesses the worth or value of an activity (by comparison with specific criteria) to support a decision or to aid an improvement. It may be a way of reducing uncertainty about the effects of continuing with an existing activity, or justifying the choice of one policy over another. Clearly establishing whether certain interventions in social work have worked or not is integral to evidence-based practice and fundamental to good practice. In addition, the receipt of funding within both the statutory and independent sector on the whole carries with it an obligation to evaluate and provide evidence of success or value for money. Evaluation may well be part of regulations and statutory requirements. Commissioners commonly use evaluation as a control measure by monitoring service activities against a specification to check that required standards have been reached.

Evaluation also has a major role in protecting the public from inappropriate or harmful practices and behind all this lies an ethical obligation to ensure that interventions are examined to make certain that they do not do any harm. Evaluators should therefore report evidence on the unintended consequences, both negative and positive, and whether short-term gains may be outweighed by long-term losses. Harmful impacts on groups indirectly affected by interventions have been proved over and over in some areas of social work; for example, in the application of legislation in the mental health field and also in the field of safeguarding vulnerable adults and children. An example of a broader evaluative approach to routine management or social work practice is the development of equality impact assessments under the Race Relations (Amendment) Act 2000 and more recently the Equality Act 2006.

Perversely, whilst evaluation is perceived to be an important aspect of performance management, it can also be seen as taking up valuable time and resources which would be better directed within highly pressurised care environments. It is therefore imperative that we are clear about whom the evaluation is for and why we are doing it. This final section of this chapter looks at why you might commission or undertake an evaluation study and the potential challenges involved. We will examine and illustrate several different approaches to evaluation and how the various stakeholders' needs are taken account of. We will cover some of the practical steps in designing and conducting an evaluation study or in your making an effective contribution to evaluation in your own organisation.

The primary purposes for evaluation

As we can see from above, those involved in commissioning or carrying out evaluations may have different purposes in mind. Green and South (2006) have summarised these as constituting four primary purposes for evaluation.

- Evaluation for accountability.
- Evaluation for learning.

- Evaluation for programme management and development.

- Evaluation as an ethical obligation.

Defining evaluation

Evaluation refers to the activity of systematically collecting, analysing and reporting information that can then be used to change attitudes or to improve the operation of a project or programme. The hallmarks of the best systematic review are explicitness and transparency and are those produced by teams comprising users, practitioners and researchers (Macdonald, 2003). Being systematic in this respect stipulates that the evaluation must be planned and have a purpose. Certain dimensions of performance such as economy, efficiency, effectiveness and ethics may be among the criteria used in the evaluation. However, evaluation goes beyond the use of information and includes feedback control. Feedback control involves using the information to make decisions about the continuation of certain practices or activities against organisational objectives. Therefore, if used effectively, evaluation is an important component of organisational learning.

Users of the evidence from evaluation will require such evidence to be robust and will expect to have a degree of confidence in the outcomes. As stated earlier, the stakeholders within the evaluation of social care will primarily be users, carers and the community, but may also involve a wide range of other stakeholders, such as policy makers and politicians, funders, managers, staff and professionals from many different disciplines, partner organisations and academics. Given that our focus in this book has been on performance management and quality assurance, we should distinguish here between evaluation and monitoring. Often when we establish a new service or project we may determine the goals or outcomes we want to achieve at the beginning and then keep track of the activities that tell us we are proceeding according to plan. What this boils down to is an emphasis on monitoring by recording what is happening as we go along. Evaluation, on the other hand, is more concerned with what has been achieved and whether and how specific changes have come about.

Who should do the evaluation?

Much of the early literature on evaluation tends to describe it as an independent and external element (Tones and Tilford, 2001), where it is seen as the preserve of professionals with specialist training. Alternatively, evaluations can be undertaken by people who are directly involved in delivering a project or service and used as internal evaluators by building on their first-hand knowledge, expertise, insight and commitment. This combats the current conceptual separation of practice information about individuals from the aggregate data required by managers for performance measurement. It militates against the notion that data for management returns are an external requirement that have little relevance to the overall business of service delivery (Gatehouse and Ward, 2003).

What are the pros and cons of these two different approaches? What do you think you would need to take into account when considering whether to commission an external evaluation or carry out an evaluation of your own service in-house?

You may wish to consider such issues as technical demands, expertise, political awareness and credibility, as well as requirements for independent scrutiny that accompany accountability for the use of public funds. The decision whether or not to commission an external evaluator may ultimately depend on the resources available, including direct and indirect costs. External evaluators are sometimes seen as more objective and impartial, particularly in relation to their independence from management and the power structures of an organisation. The other consideration is one of time availability. Ward (2004) notes the introduction of standardised formats for practitioners to record information, such as initial and core assessments designed to support the implementation of the Framework for the Assessment of Children in Need and their Families (DoH, 2000). These have meant that, at least in theory, there should be a readily accessible pool of standardised information held on all children for whom LAs hold social care responsibilities. The Integrated Children's Systems assumes that case-specific data gathered through the process of assessment, planning, intervention and review will be recorded electronically in a format that can be aggregated and used to improve services. However, according to Ward (2004), even with a fully comprehensive dataset derived from social work interactions with individual children, it seems unlikely that managers will have the time to do more than look at the surface of the information they hold in order to understand what is happening in their authority – this is where a collaborative approach, particularly in the design and strategy of an evaluation, can capitalise on both the roles of internal and external evaluators.

As we saw in Chapters 3 and 4, the importance of establishing trust and communication between those with an interest in the evaluation topic is important to its success. Likewise, successful commissioning is dependent on achieving a good fit between the purpose and scope of the evaluation and the capability of those tendering (Green and South, 2006). If you are involved in the process of commissioning, then being informed about the principles of evaluation and the implications of selecting particular research designs is essential. Clegg (2002) observed that it is common for those who are commissioning to have unrealistic expectations of what evaluators can achieve and identified the key issues as:

- modesty in expectation;

- a focus away from accountability and attribution;

- an orientation towards developing theory;

- a concern to make a reality of multi-method approaches, so that there is genuine triangulation and mutual illumination;

- an openness to complexity and systems approaches. (Clegg, 2002, cited in Green and South, 2006)

Allan (2004) talks further about the importance of being able to learn from the evaluation as a main criterion for undertaking it, and emphasises the usefulness of evaluation for constructive and critical appraisal rather than just as an affirmation of good works.

Whether commissioning an evaluation or carrying it out yourself, a number of decision-making stages needs to be followed. These will include the purpose, scope, and clarity about who the evaluation is for; ethical considerations; the design of the evaluation, i.e. what are you trying to find out; timescales and whether the information or data is accessible and available; the selection of indicators – will they actually measure what we need to measure?; the choice of data gathering methods, i.e. when will the findings be needed, where shall we gather information and how practical and cost effective are they?; the method of data analysis and interpretation; and finally, how you will present, publish and disseminate the findings and how these will be used.

Ultimately, you will need to think about the transferability of findings and their implications for practice. Findings should be contextualised appropriately and interpreted alongside other sources of evidence. If the evaluation is used to produce practice guidelines, these will inevitably have a shelf life unless they are regularly reviewed and updated. Undertaking an evaluation is not always a one-off process if its role in maintaining currency and improving quality is to be taken seriously. Once undertaken, ideally an evaluation needs to be further updated, and securing resources is another consideration in making this feasible.

Different models commonly used in evaluation

The most logical criteria to use when evaluating an intervention of any sort will relate to the goals or aims of that intervention. Goal-based evaluation focuses on the effectiveness, efficiency and economy of an intervention and can be particularly attractive if you are seeking relatively unambiguous results with clear pointers for action. It is also carried out within tight timescales and is useful where quantitative findings will be particularly valued. Taking a goal-based approach can lead to problems, however, as the goals themselves may turn out to be problematic if they are too vague or ambiguous to use as assessment criteria. A second fundamental type of problem is that goal-based evaluation may actually prevent us from identifying and evaluating most of the other effects of a programme or policy. Experts in the field of evaluation would suggest alternative approaches by distinguishing between outcome goals and activities which describe how something will be attained. Outcome goals should be clearly outcome orientated. It should be possible to know when the desired outcome has not been attained or when something else has occurred instead. Statements of goals or objectives should be also be clearly defined by avoiding jargon or buzzwords, so keep it simple. One example of a goal-based evaluation might be looking at how a community-based programme may prevent a young person from reoffending.

Illuminative evaluation is appropriate where relatively little is known about the activity you are interested in and a more exploratory approach is required. Illuminative evaluation is more concerned with checking the understanding of the situation one is in, or to reconsider working practices whose impact on goals is indirect, or to reappraise assumptions about needs or priorities in the light of new demands or unexpected difficulties. The evaluation has therefore less to do with the judgement of past performance, but more to do with people sharing their understanding of a new or difficult situation. The method of evaluation is usually qualitative but may be constrained by the cooperation or availability of those participating. When designing the evaluation study using this method, consideration needs to be given to the characteristics of the evaluator, the user, the context, the political climate and the nature and time of the report. As illuminative evaluation tends to rely on impressions, opinions and feelings, the findings may well be contested and this is commonly done by an independent evaluator. Patton (1997, p131) identifies a number of special challenges where the situation is highly-controversial. He recommends that the evaluator should have strong conflict-resolution skills and a diversity in perspective, using people management and good communication skills in order to make the best use of everyone involved. Returning to our previous example, an illuminative evaluation might seek to establish how attending a community-based programme may contribute towards a young offender's self-esteem and identity.

Economic evaluation is used to assess the relative costs and benefits of different courses of action to achieve given objectives. For example, cost-benefit analysis is a comprehensive approach that aims to clarify, quantify and value all the relevant options and their inputs and consequences. These are often expressed in monetary terms or units so that very different options can potentially be compared in the same terms. Economic evaluation techniques are relatively specialised but may not be able to address the differing values placed on inputs or outputs by stakeholders, providing instead a useful way of summarising the quantifiable impacts of care. These are used in care to help decision-makers find out whether resources are scarce and that accountability for their use needs to be shared between management, policy-makers, professionals and service users.

Accounting for every cost is a highly complex undertaking and should extend to identifying and including those besides any immediate direct costs of an intervention, such as those drawing wider sources from other agencies or the community. As economic evaluation is a specialist field, I will briefly summarise here some of the relevant models and recommend a text for further reading at the end of this chapter. Cost minimisation analysis compares the costs of alternative interventions assuming that any outcomes of each one will be the same and, on the basis of this comparison, should identify the lower-cost option. If the outcome is known to be different, or not known to be the same, then we are in the realm of cost effectiveness analysis. Here we are interested in the difference in costs between a programme and a specified alternative as a ration of the difference in outcomes (Gray, 2005a). Examples might include cost per case of population screening compared with opportunistic screening. In some circumstances, the outcome may be best measured in Quality Adjusted Life Years (QALYs). QALY economists are interested in measuring the value or utility derived from a state of well-being or change (Gray, 2005a). Cost effectiveness analysis quantifies all the costs of a project or service in monetary terms and the benefits accrued. Cost-utility analysis incorporates some consideration of the value or utility of the outcomes for example by looking at the quality of life issues. Finally, cost benefit analysis assigns costs to both the provision of an intervention and all the benefits that accrue from it. This means that these benefits must be translated into a monetary value so that the two can then be compared, often as a cost-benefit ratio. An evaluation of the cost of giving a direct payment versus the cost of providing care from an organisation to an individual would very much suit this model of evaluation, as we would also take into account the perceived choice and independence achieved in the latter process.

In some instances, discounting is used for costs over time and for those benefits which will emerge in the distant future – that is, an annual percentage reduction can be used to adjust for the declining value of money over time and the presumed lesser value of benefits (Green and South, 2006, p41). There are concerns that this favours interventions which produce outcomes relatively rapidly. Decisions about the discount rate to apply to benefits are also subjective and based on value judgements about immediate as opposed to future gains. This is a common dilemma for managers managing resource restraints and having to make decisions on a short-term basis.

Proponents of economic evaluation contend that the information it can provide is needed to make decisions about how best to allocate resources. Indeed, within cash-limited services such considerations are held to be required ethically to ensure funds are used to maximum effect. However, critics have argued that economic rationality is misplaced and concerns about such an approach range from the technical to the philosophical or ethical (Gray 2005b). Many areas of social care do not lend themselves easily to models in which there is a narrow relationship between inputs to outcomes. Godfrey (2001) notes that the principle criterion for economic evaluation is to maximise the outcomes achieved within a given budget. This might mean targeting those populations which are relatively easy to change in comparison with more challenging areas in more adverse social circumstances. Economic efficiency therefore needs to be considered alongside other such goals as equity, regeneration, social inclusion and social justice. A fundamental question is raised as to whether economic evaluation is useful and ethical in choices about the competing use of resources. You may recognise these issues from debates within the Youth Justice Service, or around the provision of certain treatments for older people, or the decision-making process around funding community-based care versus institutional care.

In conclusion, economic evaluation is a tool for making decisions about social care resources and few economists would claim that it can be used as a complete decision-making procedure. Other values, considerations and equality issues will always play a part (Gray, 2005b). But it does offer a powerful and explicit framework for considering information relevant to decision making, and as pressure on care systems increases. Economic evaluation is likely to become a more familiar and necessary tool for managers and those involved in commissioning and contracting for services. The methodology of economic evaluation is rapidly evolving. The number of economic evaluations published in the recent past have tried to reach consensus on what principles should and should not be used and clear guidelines on good practice now exist for the conduct of studies, particularly those in health economic evaluation (Gray, 2005a).

Developing evidence and indicators of quality

As we have seen, evaluation is essentially concerned with assessing whether or not interventions have been successful, and whether these have had any impact on systems and organisational developments as well as individual cases. This section is about selecting the appropriate outcome and process indicators during evaluation. Clearly, for most evaluations it is neither feasible nor desirable to measure every possible variable but we need to select indicators for capturing key aspects of the programme and its effect (Green and South, 2006). These can be quantitative – measures generated from data collected for administrative purposes which comprise aggregated data relating to a defined population at a specific point in time – or qualitative – which are more exploratory in nature and experiential. The fundamental issues are that indicators should be valid and accurately represent what they claim to represent. For example, we may have data about how many people had their needs assessed within a certain period of time and the number, type and range of services provided. Even though this data may be readily available, they cannot tell us anything about the satisfaction of service users and carers and a better indicator would involve the views of the users/carers themselves which could be obtained by using questionnaires or in-depth interviewing. In some instances, problems relating to the availability of information, measurement and data collection may make it simply not feasible to identify valid indicators. In this situation, you may need to use a proxy indicator. For example, how many people made a complaint or refused a service? The selection of indicators is ultimately influenced by values, and reflects traditional norms and managerial outcomes.

Many services focus on the achievement of more immediate outcomes rather than ultimate strategic goals. Outcome indicators need to be framed in terms of the realistic aspirations for a programme. There is frequently pressure to demonstrate outcomes that demonstrate immediate issues, for example where older people are being discharged more quickly following hospital admission to justify its existence or success. The use of intermediate indicators can help here. For example, these would occur in the causal sequence and include any of the antecedents of the outcome indicator (Green and South, 2006).

Process indicators are used to record key elements of the process of the intervention itself and contribute to the overall quality of the service. They may perhaps involve the confidence of staff that have been on a training programme and their increased involvement in raising issues at team meetings. These are sometimes also referred to as 'indirect indicators' as they are not part of the causal sequence from input to outcomes even though they contribute to the intervention itself. For example, the development of good partnerships in social care, whilst identified as a process indicator, may also prove a positive outcome in itself. Comprehensive performance assessment includes a process element by asking questions about how a local authority department promotes healthier communities or social inclusion. Understanding and articulating these different types of indicators help towards appreciating how change comes about and the complex relationships between process and outcome.

Gathering information

A key consideration in the collection of data is whether the information is fit for propose and whether it is sufficient and necessary for responding to the evaluation questions or if it needs to be supplemented in some way. In many instances, evaluation may rely on existing data and this was referred to earlier in the plethora of returns giving detail on interventions and outputs, commonly published as a series of tables and often accompanied by bulletins which gave a sophisticated analysis of trends (Ward, 2004). If your organisation employs an information officer with the necessary technical and analytical skills, you can enlist help from them. Key considerations are – who collects it, who collates it, and over what time period is it aggregated? The information you have might not be what you want, or the information you want might not be what you need and the information may be too expensive to collect within the resources available. You need to ask – what is routinely available and what will require specific data collection methods to be set up? Think about the respective responsibilities of the project and any potential in teams for data collection, particularly partnerships and co-researching opportunities with external/internal project teams to develop a process of exchange.

Evaluation or research with more hard-to-reach or marginalised groups is another challenge for agencies who are trying to promote social inclusion or diversity in service delivery. Some of the strategies recommended by Green and South (2006) include using participatory approaches which redress inequalities and minimise the power imbalances between researchers and the researched, as well as cultural and language barriers to data collection and analysis. Long-term investment in participation can build capacity in marginalised communities through developing the skills and experience of those involved (p118). They also recommend different sampling strategies such as snowball sampling, or rethinking data collection techniques by using observational methods or other media drawn from photography and videos so that they are less obtrusive yet highly visual and interactive (p122). Evaluation with hard-to-reach groups frequently involves grappling with issues around access to services in the first place and one of the aims of any evaluation should be to help shed light on inequalities in provision and gather evidence to help address these. Illuminative evaluation and a human rights approach can provide a mechanism for delivering genuine accountability in performance measurement.

ACTIVITY **5.2**

You could try to put into practice some of the suggestions above by thinking about what methods might be appropriate to assess the provision of a service in your specialisms for a particular minority group.

Taking up the challenge – developing evidence-based practice

In Chapter 3 we looked at leadership and organisational culture. Leadership is seen as one of a number of related factors which are reported as supporting the use of evidence in practice and the effective uptake of research evidence (Kitson et al., 1998). Line managers are by far the most frequently cited source of support for practitioners, yet many managers express their own lack of confidence in this area and describe their role predominantly in terms of directing staff to other resources (Buxton et al., 1998). A review of the literature on leading evidence-informed practice (Research in Practice, 2003) distinguishes a number of people as having a role in leading evidence-informed practice. These are operational managers derived from their formal positions of authority; opinion leaders who because of their status or technical competence are able to influence other individuals' attitudes or overt behaviour informally in a desired way with relative frequency (Kitson et al., 1998); facilitators who are external experts in the management of change and who consciously use a series of interpersonal and group skills to help people change their habits, skills, ways of thinking and working and can overcome favourable, contextual conditions (Kitson et al., 1998); and product or issue 'champions' or change agents, who as identifiable enthusiasts, have credibility in the organisation and can act as a catalyst for promoting the integration of available research into policy and practice (Hughes and Traynor, 2000). Finally, Percy-Smith (2002) in her report on research in local government recognises the important role of elected members, particularly their scrutiny role. The Cabinet Office Performance and Innovation Unit (2000) report also highlights the role of elected members in establishing appropriate values (all cited in Research in Practice, 2003).

Table 5.1 below summarises the functions of leaders of evidence-informed practice beginning with relaying evidence and monitoring its implementation, nurturing and facilitating staff within their own areas of practice, and direct role modelling (Research in Practice, 2003).

Table 5.1 A summary of the functions of leaders of evidence-informed practice

Setting direction and expectation	1. debating what being 'evidence-informed' means in terms of policy and practice
	2. articulating a clear vision and set of values about EIP to guide individual actions
	3. developing a plan showing how EIP will be taken forward, including identifying leaders or champions
	4. monitoring progress with the plan and revising it accordingly
	5. talking to practitioners about the importance, benefits and ethics of understanding and using evidence, and creating an expectation that it will happen
	6. identifying and addressing resistance to change (e.g. through incentives)

Increasing the competence of staff	7. analysing the development needs of individuals with regard to finding, appraising, using and generating evidence, and setting related objectives
	8. identifying and using appropriate methods to meet these development needs
	9. regularly discussing progress against developmental objectives and reviewing achievements
	10. preventing decay in professional knowledge/expertise and ensuring practitioners keep up to date (e.g. through professional meetings and peer discussions to critically review new evidence)
	11. providing opportunities for continuing professional development to expose staff to different perspectives on practice (e.g. courses, study, research)
Supporting and enabling critical thinking about practice	12. communicating relevant evidence to staff
	13. spending time with others reflecting on established procedures and past experiences/events (such as visits, assessments, interventions, incidents) and raising questions about decisions, plans and results
	14. creating the conditions in which learning can occur (e.g. setting broad objectives and constraints, ensuring working practices are flexible enough to allow change and providing time for practitioners to debate practice issues)
	15. harnessing objective outside views to generate insights (e.g. from new staff, students or external agencies)
	16. identifying where more detailed investigations, reviews of evidence, formal research or evaluation will have maximum impact
Using evidence to improve services for users	17. piloting/trialling new ideas where there is a clear evidence base
	18. implementing relevant findings by incorporating them in work practices, procedures and processes
	19. managing the implications and risks of changing practices (e.g. staff motivation when preferred ways of working are not supported by best available evidence or professional judgements are challenged)
Generating and sharing evidence	20. promoting the systematic collection and comparative analysis of data about performance
	21. establishing monitoring, self-audit and feedback mechanisms
	22. encouraging reviews of evidence, formal research, evaluation of practice and listening to users to generate knowledge
	23. supporting the research activities of staff and their involvement in studies
	24. sharing learning with others (e.g. by presenting and publishing interesting cases, small-scale evaluations, reports of innovations and records of reflection on practice to a wider audience)
Modelling appropriate behaviour	25. demonstrating awareness of best available evidence in the field
	26. showing an understanding of current research and its nature and limitations
	27. taking action to ensure that effective use is made of relevant evidence and research
	28. basing own decisions on a proper consideration of the evidence
	29. asking what the evidence is to support a policy change (or no change)
	30. challenging assumptions and mental models to allow new ideas to be conceived and alternative working methods to be considered
	31. establishing outcome measures and targets for teams
	32. using evidence about outcomes and targets to manage performance

Creating strategic
partnerships

33. involving internal people who can facilitate or support EIP (e.g. trainers, practice teachers, IT)

34. building close ties with local and national education/ research establishments

35. securing funding to invest in EIP (e.g. training/education of practitioners, sources of evidence, information systems)

36. liaising with external people and agencies who can support EIP and to share learning

37. rewarding good practice

Reproduced by kind permission of *Research in Practice* which is part of the Dartington Hall Trust. The above abstract has subsequently been published in the *Leading Evidence Informed Handbook*; see Hodson R (2003) *A Review of Literature on Leading Evidence Informed Practice*, Research in Practice – further useful resources can be found in Hodson, R and Cooke, E (2007) *Leading Evidence Informed Practice Research in Practice*. www.rip.org.uk/publications/handbooks.asp

C H A P T E R   S U M M A R Y

In this chapter, we began by considering the usefulness of evidence and research in social care and their potential contribution to developing quality care or improving quality and concluded that this is a controversial area. Managing quality requires the active management of different types of knowledge and the process of its acquisition and dissemination in order to inform and improve practice. We have noted the importance of having clear objectives in the first place and establishing appropriate measures and indicators using the example of undertaking an evaluation study. Having a model for thinking about evaluation requires making a connection between services and an existing evidence base and can give service design a renewed focus (Axford et al., 2005). The selection of methods for measuring outcomes and process should be based on a consideration of reliability, validity, suitability for purpose, feasibility, consistency with the values of work on the project and appropriateness for use with other groups (Green and South, 2006). The question of what supports or hinders the translation of policy vision into practical reality is pivotal for the role of leaders in practice environments, and you may wish to consider and develop your own competence in this area to equip you with the confidence, skills and knowledge to develop this in your team and service areas.

FURTHER READING

Department of Health (2005c) *Research governance framework for health and social care.* The second edition of this framework outlines the principles of good governance that apply to all research in relation to good practice and risk-based regulatory process. It applies to the full range of research types, contexts and methods and the interest of research participants is enshrined in the guidance. Available from **www.dh.gov.uk/publications/guidance**

Drummond, F, Torrance, G W, O'Brien, B, J and Sculpher, M (2005) *Methods for the Economic Evaluation of Health Care Programmes.* Oxford: Oxford University Press
This is a standard textbook used by those undertaking economic evaluation in health and outlines the key methodological principles using practical exercises. It is adaptable for those working in multi-disciplinary teams or commissioners interested in or needing to find out more about these approaches.

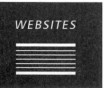

WEBSITES

www.rip.org.uk *Research in Practice* is the largest children and families' research implementation project in England and Wales and aims to promote and disseminate evidence-informed practice across a broad membership by using a variety of methods at many organisational levels.

www.evidencenetwork.org/ *ESRC Evidence Network* provides a focal point for those interested in evidence-based policy and practice and supplies a forum for debate, discussion and dissemination on evidenced-based issues. You can join the network through the website.

www.scie.org.uk Social Care Institute for Excellence's aim is to improve the experience of people who use social care by developing and promoting knowledge about good practice in the sector. Using knowledge gathered from diverse sources and a broad range of people and organisations, SCIE develops and shares resources such as systematic knowledge reviews, guidance and position papers, all of which are available free via the website.

Chapter 6
Improving quality through supporting the workforce

ACHIEVING POST-QUALIFYING SOCIAL WORK AWARDS

If you are a registered social worker, this chapter will assist you to evidence post-registration training and learning. It relates to the national post-qualifying framework for social work education and training, in particular the national criteria at the higher specialist/advanced level.
- *iv Demonstrate a fully developed capacity to take responsibility for the use of reflection and critical analysis to continuously develop and improve own performance and the performance of professional and interprofessional groups, teams and networks in the context of professional practice, professional management, professional education or applied professional research,*

The leadership and management standards in social care
- *D2 Develop productive working relationships with colleagues and stakeholders*
- *D4 Plan the workforce – taking a lead in identifying the workforce requirements of your organisation and how these will be satisfied.*
- *D6 Provide learning opportunities for colleagues to improve performance with emphasis on developing a learning culture with the organisation so that colleagues take responsibility for their own learning and are supported in this by the organisation.*

Introduction

Workforce planning and workforce development are relatively new areas in social work and social care and present us with a number of challenges and difficulties. Within the ever-evolving policy environment, growing expectations from service users and society, demographic challenges and new technologies within an environment of economic restraints, it is clear that analysing and maximising the use of current and future resources, particularly human resources, are essential to provide quality services (Scottish Workforce Unit, 2006, p4). Estimates suggest that over a million people are employed in the social care sector, one third of whom are employed by local authorities in England (Local Authority Workforce Intelligence Group, 2006), and the remaining two thirds are working in the independent sector (Moriarty, 2004). The emphasis on regulation, registration and upskilling of the workforce within the sector demands a clear action plan for supporting and developing human resources in order to achieve organisational goals and to deliver flexible and responsive services.

This is not without its contradictions, as for some time now there has been concern that social work is a 'demographic time bomb' in terms of the nature of the qualified workforce (McLenachan, 2006). In social care, many staff are now nearing retirement, leaving some agencies concerned about losing significant numbers of their qualified and experienced workforce over the next decade. Continuing themes relating to workforce capacity remain related to not only age profiles, but also to gender, ethnicity, career progression and job satisfaction. Recent government recruitment campaigns have targeted social work and social care in an attempt to encourage people to consider this as a worthwhile career (*www.socialworkandsocialcare.co.uk*). These campaigns operate in the context of sometimes negative images being portrayed in the media about social work in particular and also showing demonisation of the people workers help. These pose really major stumbling blocks to addressing workforce development issues. Discrepancies in pay and status have also been highlighted by social workers within inter-professional teams, reinforcing the view that their professional status and the social work role are together less valued and respected (McLenachan, 2006).

This chapter will go on to look at some of the strategic drivers for workforce planning and development and will address a few of the specific areas within your own teams and services where you could have a direct impact on supporting the workforce to respond appropriately to these demands. We will start with an overview of the main drivers for workforce development and then go on to look at specific issues such as supervision, promoting diversity in workforce development, the practical challenges for supporting staff in the face of stress and the need for developing competence at work.

Workforce planning – a toolkit

Good quality information about supply, recruitment and retention is essential in providing an evidence base for planning workforce development (Moriarty, 2004). Workforce planning is a collaborative process which can take place at different levels within the organisation and using input from different people. The Scottish Workforce Unit (2006) for the voluntary sector in Scotland has provided a helpful toolkit which spells out the various steps involved in workforce planning and is structured around six key stages:

1. Getting started by establishing scope, timescales and deciding who should be involved.

2. Considering the organisational context for developing a workforce plan and the external drivers that impact on planning and delivering your service particularly for the future.

3. Building a picture of the workforce by gathering data about numbers and roles of staff, their levels of knowledge, skills and exact qualifications. Undertaking regular training needs analysis which should also cover other functions such as health and safety, mentoring and CPD requirements, and to particularly note specific skills brought into the organisation by other members of the workforce.

4. Developing a vision for the future by blending the ideal with a realistic picture of where your service is actually going. This process should involve consultation and visioning exercises with staff and service users to encourage creativity and joined-up thinking between partnerships or units. Key priorities can be identified from your business, corporate and service plans as well as by taking a thorough look at current work practices and skills mix. Being aware of regulatory requirements alongside funding and resources is important for planning purposes.

5. Analysing any gaps or surpluses in your workforce should enable you to identify priority areas for development when developing plans and strategies to bridge the gap. Two main options for bridging gaps include planning to support, develop and retain existing staff and recruiting new members to your workforce through redesign of new roles. The National Occupations Standards can be a useful tool when assessing job roles and specification. Succession and career planning for existing staff are useful for linking the learning and development needs of the current workforce with future skills gaps and utilising opportunities such as secondments or job shadowing within the organisation.

6. Developing and evaluate your workforce plan and keeping it under regular review. (*Reprinted with kind permission of the Scottish Workforce Unit www.workforce.org.uk*)

In the human resources literature, workforce development is often linked to successful business strategies and performance improvement. Table 6.1 on p108 summarises the business case for workforce planning and the benefits for different stakeholders to which you could add any of your own imperatives.

A profile of the social care workforce in the UK tells us that women make up the majority, ranging from 80.6 per cent in England (Local Authority Workforce Intelligence Group, 2006) to 90 per cent in Scotland and 95 per cent in Northern Ireland (Moriarty, 2004). The proverbial glass ceiling remains with women comprising the majority of home care staff, residential workers, field social workers and managers, but with under-representation in senior positions and a higher rate of part-time working. Staff in an NISW study (2000) revealed that care workers were not as interested in acquiring a qualification as in undertaking training which took account of their family circumstances, previous educational experience and learning styles. Staff particularly wanted training to support their direct work in specialist areas. The NISW study also found that higher proportions of staff working with children and families tend to have professional qualifications. Staff going on to do social work qualifications after working in residential care could be an important resource in increasing the overall pool of social workers, as staff training through employment-based routes were found to be more likely to remain working with the same employer or user group in the longer term.

The social care workforce as a whole is predominantly female; 80 per cent increasing to 95 per cent in certain sectors such as residential, domiciliary care and some areas of early years. Mainly as a consequence of this, nearly 50 per cent of the workforce work part-time (Skills for Care, 2004a). Annual turnover for all directly employed staff in social services in England at the end of September was 11 per cent with higher turnover rates in the South East of up to 17.5 per cent (Skills for Care, 2004a) and younger staff staying for shorter periods, and male managers staying on for longer (McLean and Andrew, 1998). In relation to commitment, organisational research suggests that this has a greater influence on job performance and service quality than job satisfaction and also has an affective dimension. McLean (2002) found a distinction between staff's commitment to an organisation and commitment to their profession (where managers and social workers were more likely to have affective commitment to the

Table 6.1 The business case for workforce planning

Benefits for employers	Benefits for members of the organisation	Benefits for service users
Maximises potential of the current workforce	Helps to maximise staff potential and the development of knowledge, skills and competencies	Well-trained and competent staff who are always looking to develop their skills
Helps to achieve regulatory requirements		
Enables identification of current skills gaps and appropriate responses	Stable teams, fuller employment and less stress on existing staff	More stability in relationships with staff with less turnover
Helps predict and plan for future skills, service needs and gaps	Succession planning and career development	Continuity in care in staff training and learning which has an impact on the design and delivery of the services wanted and needed.
Facilitates effective bidding for resources	Job satisfaction	
Links learning and development with service needs	Encourages and contributes to the development of continuous improvement and the quality of service delivered	
Helps maximise the use of technology and new practice ideas		
Improves staff retention through support, learning and development, and career pathways		
Reduces recruitment and turnover costs		
Improves service delivery		
Creates sustainable services capable of responding to changing needs and demands on the workforce		

Source: Scottish Workforce Unit (2006) With thanks to the Voluntary Sector Social Services Workforce Unit (Scotland) for permission to reproduce this information.

latter). Direct care workers, however, showed greater commitment to the organisation or service setting and therefore tended to give longer service.

Supporting your workforce

The above data have important implications for recruitment and retention policies, suggesting that familiarity with issues in your workforce underpins the potential to improve commitment, job satisfaction and job control and to reduce work related stress by giving attention to the immediate work environment (Moriarty, 2004). Ongoing reforms in the social care workforce have sought to establish career pathways across health and social care in adult services, and a shared set of skills, knowledge and behaviours for those working within integrated services. Developing the needs of professionals from different backgrounds with varying levels of responsibility and from a range of settings will affect senior professionals developing integrated commissioning, those individuals working in partnerships with the voluntary and community sector. It will also affect workers serving the specific groups of service users with specialist and complex needs, including early intervention and prevention and within co-located or virtual teams with members from a number of different agencies (DfES, 2005b). As career pathways change over time, it is likely that there will also be more overlap with different professional groups. Some of the new challenges managers are likely to face are a much greater knowledge requirement of different legal and policy frameworks as well as individual team members' expertise, the need to provide adequate cover for colleagues in small multi-disciplinary teams and ensuring individuals feel confident and competent enough to take on new roles and responsibilities. Following from our discussion in Chapter 4, managers will also need to manage the transition from a provider-led approach, to one where users and carers are increasingly empowered to be partners in determining priorities (DfES, 2005b). These demands inevitably link to your own continuing professional development needs so that you are able to translate strategic vision into local plans in collaboration with professionals, partners and users.

ACTIVITY 6.1

The above agenda represents a tall order for leaders and managers and is linked to the increasing emphasis on management development programmes in social care. Take a few minutes to consider which specific roles and functions you have in developing staff for whom you have responsibility. Identify any specific areas of your own knowledge or skills which need to be improved. Who can help you with these and what additional resources might you require i.e time, people, money, specialist training, information, etc.?

Lessons learnt from implementing new ways of working have shown that one of the major facilitators of change is to establish and foster a learning culture. According to Walton (2005), a learning culture in its wider context is one which enables the liberation of learning from the political and administrative preoccupations of central government. It facilitates the connection between extending and disseminating knowledge to maintain and improve the standards of practice and consciously develops opportunities to work on partnerships which will provide support for the expansion of staff development and opportunities for practitioner involvement in organisational development and the provision of high quality services. As we saw in the previous chapter, good staff development and a sense of being valued by employers are crucial to promoting an environment in which staff feel able to manage their work, and where the chance to enhance the knowledge and skills needed to keep pace with changes in legislation, policy and the research context of practice exists. Creating conditions that promote ethical reflections on practice must start with robust supervision arrangements and it is to this area which we will now turn.

Supervision

Social work supervision has been identified as one of the most significant factors in determining the job satisfaction levels of front-line social workers and has been cited as a crucial determinant of service quality (Morrison, 2002).

> *This inquiry saw too many examples of those in senior positions attempting to justify their work in terms of bureaucratic activity rather than outcomes for people.* (Lord Laming at the Victoria Climbié Inquiry)

Being a supervisor will allow you to increase your own development skills in helping others to learn and develop within their work, as well as offering a chance to use your own experience to help supervisees develop their own style of working and find their own solutions to difficult problems. Supervision has been a core activity for social work and social care in the last decade, particularly given the focus on public enquiries which has raised its profile largely from a defensive perspective (Morrison, 2002). As a pivotal activity in delivering social care services, supervision is the key to achieving quality assurance, but has a particular role in developing a skilled and professional workforce. Professional supervision provides a bridge between first line managers and practitioners. Hawkins and Shoet (2006, p50), building on work done by Gilbert and Evans (2000), list what they feel are the essential qualities of effective supervisors.

- Flexibility in moving between theoretical concepts and the use of a wide variety of interventions and methods.

- A multi-perspectival view in being able to see the same situation from a variety of angles.

- A working map of the discipline in which they supervise.

- The ability to work transculturally.

- The capacity to manage and contain anxiety both their own and that of the supervisee.

- Openness to learning from supervisees and from new situations that emerge.

- Sensitivity to the wider contextual issues that impact on both the therapeutic and supervisory processes.

- Handling power appropriately and in a non-oppressive way.

- Having humour, humility and patience.

From a supervisee's point of view, the objectives of supervision are to improve a worker's capacity to do the job effectively by providing a good work environment, professional knowledge, practice skills, and emotional support. The ultimate objective is to provide effective and efficient service to users by ensuring the satisfactory job performance and professional competence of front-line staff. Therefore supervision is an important and integral component of any practice in social care (Morrison, 2002).

Good supervision inevitably focuses some attention on the dynamics of the process but these must arise out of work-related issues and be done to enable the supervisee to manage the work better. Within the context of quality and performance management, supervision is often vertical, by which is meant you will work as a more experienced supervisor with a less experienced supervisee. Within the multi-disciplinary environment, different types of supervision models may be more appropriate, for example as a form of consultancy, peer or group supervision which starts from a sharing of mutual expectations and will require the fostering of trust, goodwill and respect between all the parties concerned. Potential value conflicts with other professions require the exploration and recognition of the values of various organisational participants, both within and between professions. Where a clear policy for inter-professional supervision does not exist, it is important to clarify the professional and ethical codes of conduct from each professional and the boundaries involved. Group supervision, combined with individual supervision, has several advantages besides economies of scale; it can develop a supportive atmosphere between peers thus reducing dependency and providing a wider range of knowledge, skills and expertise. From the perspective of the service user, interprofessional work can facilitate the bringing together of skills and information that provide continuity in care and the apportionment of clear responsibilities and accountabilities (Townend, 2005).

Research has described managers as not only the most stressed workers within a social services department, but also the ones who consider themselves least well-prepared and supported in doing their current job (Balloch et al., 1995). Lack of attention to your own supervision needs can lead to poor communication, a fragmentation of the decision-making process and a defensive retreat. The first step to becoming a skilled supervisor is to receive good supervision yourself. Supervision training for all staff throughout an organisation using workshops and conferences as well as formal training courses and CPD can provide an impetus for raising the level of supervision practice. In conclusion, whether your supervision relationships within multi-disciplinary groups are peer-led or part of a working team, their effectiveness will depend to a large extent on the ability of members to be aware of, and to process, any group dynamics that prevail. Training for managers that enables them to also take on the role of educator within the supervision or team/group contexts should also be supplemented by regular updates on research and promote a culture of reflection within the profession which will stimulate and promote the desire to know more (Hafford-Letchfield et al., 2007).

The quality of supervision depends on several factors including the relationships between individual parties and the contract, format and developmental stages of the supervisory process. Hawkins and Shoet (2006, p61) offer the following basic guidelines in their CLEAR model (Contract, Listen, Explore, Action and Review) as a starting point for supervision (and which I have expanded upon).

- Developing a contract – supervision should start with establishing the supervisee's desired outcomes, understanding what needs to be covered and how the process can be most valuable. This includes agreeing any basic groundrules or roles. Build on any supervision policies and pro-formas available to ensure that agency standards are met.

- Active listening and catalytic interventions to promote understanding of the situation in which the supervisee wants to make a difference – supervisors need to express accurate empathy through reframing, drawing on evidence, theory or research in order to make new connections with what has been shared.

- Exploring through questioning, reflection and generation of new insight and awareness so that supervisors work with the supervisee in partnership to envision different options for handling the issues.

- Taking action – having explored the various dynamics and scenarios within the situation and developed different options for handling it, the supervisee is encouraged to choose a way forward and agrees the first steps. At this point it may be helpful to rehearse any strategies together and check for any new learning needs that should be met in order to deal with the situation effectively.

- Review the actions that have been agreed – the supervisor should encourage feedback from the supervisee on what was helpful about the supervision process and what was difficult and how future working relationships can be improved. Agreeing and documenting a plan of action for review at future supervision sessions completes the work.

It is not possible to overstate the importance of good regular and planned supervision. In social care organisations, the approach to supervision can often reflect the level of control exercised by the agency. Morrison (2002) describes these two extremes, the first is the casework model which is based on a high level of administrative accountability fitting with well-documented managerialist approaches. At the other extreme is the autonomous practice model where there is a high level of professional autonomy. Supervisors can act as change agents by using their 'go-between' role with senior management and front-line staff, as well as have an advocate role to protect and assert the rights of staff. This involves developing an awareness of your own power and authority in the supervisory relationship and working towards ethical management practice. Administrative authority is frequently easily accepted by supervisees and this is where dignity-at-work issues begin to surface. Approaches to team working and fostering learning cultures as explored in Chapter 3 can help in this area. In summary, monitoring professional performance and the quality of practice through supervision refers to the application of professional values, knowledge and skills which can also be acquired and validated through the educative function of the supervision process. Attention to the learning of supervisees and their lifelong learning needs, and aligning these with organisational goals by providing opportunities to do so, can motivate staff to achieve a higher level of job performance.

Wellbeing at work and supporting staff through difficulties

In Chapter 3 we looked at the concept of emotional intelligence, how this is considered important within a leadership role and the impact of emotions and feelings on the culture of the workplace. Reflecting upon effective social work interventions in complex care settings is important within supervision and the day-to-day context in social work and social care. According to Morrison (2007), there will always be some staff who may be struggling or will be at 'borderline' levels of competence, despite the provision of more supportive arrangements, and who find reflection difficult or experience problems in taking into sufficient account the views, wishes or feelings of users and colleagues. Referring to his own experiences as a mentor for managers and supervisors dealing with difficult staff management situations, Morrison suggests that the most troubling and intractable situations exist when performance difficulties occur in the context of staff who lack accurate empathy, self-awareness and self-management skills.

> *This lack of emotional competence renders the specific performance problems such as poor recording practice, all but unmanageable. In the worst cases, these become almost 'toxic' in such a way that whole teams or even agencies can become enmeshed in the distorting dynamics surrounding the individual staff member.* (Morrison, 2007, p247)

It is clear then, that the handling of emotion and the process of care are inextricably connected to the quality of care. Unless such expert or intuitive practice can be described and articulated through the process of critical reflection and within a culture of learning, the pursuit of pure technical competencies in which expertise is neither described nor valued will prevail (Benner, 2001).

UK social research and international comparators consistently profile the social care profession as one where there are high levels of stress, sickness absence and burnout (Stanley et al., 2007). Various studies on these issues within the workforce have found that the highest level of mental health problems are amongst those working in children's services (Bennet et al., 1993). A postal survey of 1,000 social workers in the USA (Siebert, 2004, cited in Stanley et al., 2007) found that 19 per cent scored above the threshold on the Centre for Epidemiologic Studies–Depression Scale, with 20 per cent taking medication. Sixty per cent considered that they were or had been depressed, with an alarming 16 per cent of respondents having seriously considered suicide at some point. Stanley et al. (2007) made their own study of depression in the social work profession and found that work played a substantial part in its development. High demands, a perceived lack of control and an absence of boundaries, whether in relation to the size of the workload or the distressing nature of the work, were highlighted as relevant (p293). Stanley et al. also found that middle management was no more immune to the experiences of depression than their colleagues. The experience of work as excessively demanding was not just a matter of volume, but some of those interviewed in the study had also downgraded to a post without management responsibilities to avoid high levels of responsibility, as well as other social workers moving into management roles to escape face-to-face work with service users (Stanley et al., 2007). The impact of technology has introduced teleworking to social care where employees work outside the workplace using electronic communication which has strengthened certain aspects and dimensions of social work services. The use of such technology can also be exploited when used to intrude into staff personal time at home where the boundaries are unclear. Its further use in monitoring worker productivity can also dominate other means of communication and workload management.

Mechanisms for protecting staff from these kinds of pressures could include realistic workload management systems, regular supervision and contact with colleagues which has been shown to be one of the most rewarding and protective elements of the job (Reid et al., 1999). Staff may not always be able to recognise their own stress and reactions to work, and many studies have found that disclosure is experienced as problematic at a number of levels because of the stigmatising effect and the intolerant culture in the workplace. Stanley et al.'s (2007) study cited colleagues' attitudes and support as very relevant to recovery and the attitudes of managers and human resource staff as a significant factor in determining the nature and extent of adaptations offered to staff experiencing mental health problems. Developing policies in the workplace that support a work-life balance i.e. home working, flexibility for families and carers, for example through flexible leave arrangement, and subsidised leisure facilities, can all help to reduce workplace stress and support staff in working to their full potential. A report by the Joint Review Team (Audit Commission, 2002) highlighted five issues consistently identified as being most important to staff. These were: feeling they are making a positive difference to service users' lives; being clear about what is expected of them and being given constructive feedback; having attention paid to their personal development; having a voice in the organisation; having fair workloads and terms and conditions.

Diversity and fairness in the workplace

Changing demographics and the process of globalisation have made diversity in organisations responsible for delivering social care services a major focal point. All of the existing data indicate that, if diversity is the issue, then inclusion is the answer – one that focuses on management practices and organisational systems that maximise the contribution of all employees in the workforce (Giovannini, 2004). Managing diversity effectively among employees is a complex area posing many challenges and opportunities for social care managers. Effective management of diversity has moral, ethical and social dimensions. It must meet legal requirements and is directly related to quality and performance issues in service delivery (Taylor (1993) cited in Lymbery, 2001). This concerns not only the inclusion and support of staff from different backgrounds, but also that the skills and knowledge of all staff should be able to provide effective services to the community and to develop cultural competence.

Leadership is required in identifying, redressing and eliminating gaps and deficiencies in cross-cultural knowledge and standards for professional competence within the organisation, alongside the commitment of resources to achieve this (Malcolm, 2007). In addition, in the context of social care (and allied professions), there has been a widespread recognition that implementing anti-discriminatory practice and promoting diversity are key components of leadership and management tasks. However, what is less convincing is the ability of leaders and managers to incorporate diversity and proactively tackle discrimination through the process of facilitating learning and development (Begum, 2007). Much of the diversity management literature places a strong emphasis on improving corporate performance and creating more socially inclusive work environments by *releasing desperately needed talents suppressed by mono-cultural organisations that label and stereotype on the basis of race, sexuality, disability and so on* (Lorbiecki, 2001, p346). Whilst much of the focus within organisations has been on equipping managers to tackle discrimination and promote diversity, there is now a growing acknowledgement that supporting learning and development has to be explicitly at the core of promoting diversity (Begum, 2007).

Pelmutter et al. (2001), cited in Malcolm (2007, p133), discuss three theoretical orientations to diversity in the workplace; legal, which emphasises knowledge about and adherence to the law; anthropological, which centres on an awareness of cultures; and finally the socio-psychological, which focuses on diversity as in differences and similarities between individuals, groups, organisational values, knowledge and skills. Malcolm asserts that social work and social care managers must have knowledge and skills spanning all three orientations, where organisational efforts aimed at valuing diversity must include the structural as well as the social if true multiculturalism is to be achieved (p133).

Diversity in workforce development – some of the issues

Equal opportunities and diversity in workforce development have been issues of long-standing concern within both the health and social care sector (King's Fund, 1990; DoH, 2001a, 2005c). According to Friday and Friday (2003) managing diversity is an active management process to direct what individuals bring to the organisation to help it meet its strategic goals. Redressing the balance of women, minority and ethnic group representation at all levels of employment in the sector has also been linked to social inclusion strategies (Davidson, 1997; ADSS, 2004). So bridging any gulf between the espoused commitments of an organisation and having an agenda for action can contribute towards the delivery of accessible, high-quality services. However, simply recruiting people from different backgrounds is not enough; there has to be a complementary effort to support those individuals once they have entered the organisation and to provide a supportive environment (Johns and Jordan, 2006).

Research into diversity management demonstrates under- and over-representation of some groups in social care employment and the nature of the discrimination they experience. For example, findings suggest that black and minority ethnic managers received less supervisory support, training and development opportunities, and high quality feedback than other managers (Improvement and Development Agency, 2004), and are more likely to miss important developmental opportunities to aid their career progression. Whilst these findings relate to senior managers, it is clear that management development structures are required at all levels in an organisation, in a way that is transparent, fair and consistent (Hafford-Letchfield and Chick, 2006c).

For learners, social work education is not immune to challenges to widening partici- pation. In 2005, the GSCC documented issues regarding progression rates for black, minority and disabled candidates. A commissioned study demonstrated that social work students from black and minority ethnic groups were less likely to progress in time than white students, irrespective of such factors as age or gender (GSCC and King's College, 2006). The reasons for this were cited as *complicated and likely to relate not only to the characteristics of individual students but also to the university in which they study* (GSCC, 2005, p11). The number of black social workers varies greatly geographically but in 2004, 82 per cent of social services was reported to be white with one black social services director in 2003. Evidence that black and minority ethnic staff tend be more qualified that their white counterparts indicates that the nature of the barriers they face needs to be addressed. Various studies have documented the racist behaviour towards black staff from service users, their relatives and colleagues (Moriarty, 2004; Butt and Davey, 1997). The forms this behaviour took were varied and ranged from verbal abuse and physical violence to more covert instances, such as the undermining of people at work (Moriarty, 2004). Whilst all staff can experience violence at work, any racist or homophobic elements to violence can be most promi- nent in front-line work. Staff in some studies have reported a lack of confidence in the ability of their managers and employers to take sufficient action (Butt and Davey, 1997; Butt, 2005). This emphasises the need for managers and employers to take a more proactive role in tackling the issues of racism and heterosexism in the workplace.

Beyond the proverbial 'glass ceiling', various determinants, particularly institutional bar- riers, continue to affect disadvantaged groups' access to career progression (Liff and Dale, 1994; Harlow, 2004). The census shows that some gains have been made by women who now hold about a third of managerial jobs in the UK, mostly in occupation subgroups in the public sector such as finance, office, health and social care manage- ment (Equal Opportunities Commission, 2003) but women make up only 16 per cent of local authority leaders (*The Guardian*, 2006). The government recently launched an action plan to close the gender pay gap. Creating more quality part-time roles is key to increasing the number of women in senior positions, which can extend an agency's portfolio of skills and provide role models for younger and aspiring women with poten- tial. The work/home-life conflict can be one barrier to women seeking promotion to management positions, particularly at senior levels (Harlow, 2004), due to unresponsive cultures and a lack of robust work-life policies (Bryans and Mavin, 2003).

The Disability Discrimination Act 1995 focused employers' attention on the issue of discrimination against disabled people in the workplace. According to Moriarty (2004) data collected by independent researchers are of particular value because many work- ers are reluctant to discuss their health with their employers for fear that they will be stigmatised or that their career prospects will be affected. The cost implications of provision for employees with disabilities or fears about them requiring a lot of sickness absence have been shown to be unfounded. Employers do need to consider solutions, such as flexible working patterns that will lessen the impact of the work culture or environment on people with disabilities and must ensure that there are confidential procedures by which people can discuss issues relating to their health and work without compromising their privacy or confidentiality.

References to men working in social care are rarely made except in terms of this being a non-traditional area of paid male employment, and the literature on this topic tends to lack an empirical base. The workforce data suggest that while men form a small proportion of the total social care workforce they are concentrated in certain areas, such as working with children, adolescents or adults with a mental health or learning disability (Moriarty, 2004). Among senior managers men are in the majority, and in comparison only a fifth of black men are in managerial posts (*The Guardian*, 2006). One of the explanations given for this is that men in caring and related occupations often refer to mixed responses from other people about their choice of employment, and feeling pressurised to seek managerial posts (Moriarty, 2004).

Heterosexism in the workplace can manifest itself in a number of different forms and is often based on the belief that heterosexuality is the only normal, valid, and moral basis for a lifestyle. The degree to which this attitude is present in the work environment varies. There may be some workplaces where prejudice and discrimination against lesbian, gay and bisexual workers have been infrequently challenged in the past. Changing the heterosexist culture requires social care organisations and providers to demonstrate strong but sensitive leadership. Managers will need to give consideration to how the work environment could be improved to provide a safe and supportive place for staff and service users to 'come out' – the decision about whether or not to 'come out' is a difficult and ongoing process for many LGBT people, who have to continuously weigh up the risks and benefits of telling others about their sexual orientation. This may include a consideration of possible reactions from service users and a fear of detrimental effects on career advancement or career options. Not being 'out' at work can create additional stress and anxiety for staff already in stressful job. If they fear a homophobic reaction, or that people will not be comfortable with their sexual orientation, they will edit what they disclose about their personal life, their partner, or even where they go and what they do socially. This can lead eventually to feelings of isolation and maybe even withdrawal from the normal 'banter' which can occur in the workplace (www.pace.org.uk).

Johns and Jordan (2006) have argued that the goal of diversity in recruitment (and retention) for professional work *cannot easily be reconciled with the narrow, traditional interpretation of social work as competent casework, or the highly individualistic version of service delivery, choice and citizenship which the New Labour government applies to social care* (p1273). They recommend adopting a far broader perspective on the values, goals and merits of people from a diverse range of backgrounds, valuing them on the basis of their group identities and personal experiences. Whether positive action can drive forward equality of opportunity is debatable, as it guarantees only equality of competition without necessarily changing outcomes (Hafford-Letchfield and Chick, 2006; Johns and Jordan, 2006). Lorbiecki's (2001) learning model approach, as the name suggests, is constructed on the notion that individuals and organisations have to recognise that diversity is a multifaceted social construction. It is a complex phenomenon which *sees people not in terms of what they look like, or where they come from, but through incorporating their different, important and competitively relevant knowledge and perspectives about how to actually do the work which is learnt from the experience of being members of different groups* (p346). There is no standard prescription for managing diversity except that you must create a climate in which initiatives around diversity can flourish and encourage cultural change through promoting learning from both internal and external evidence-based practice (Singh, 2002). Ensuring that the different strands of equality and anti-discriminatory elements (age, race, religion, sexual orientation, disability, gender) are addressed within broader based diversity approaches requires careful attention so that the experiences and concerns of staff emerging from the different forms of oppression are not diluted or overlooked (Begum, 2007).

Formal and informal learning can encourage staff to participate in debates about diversity in your service. Solutions might include developing positions in which the roles of practitioners and manager are less apparent or divisive, and encouraging more dialogue so that staff can learn from each other's perspectives. To encourage succession planning and remove barriers to career progression and personal and professional development, the use of shadowing, mentoring and coaching schemes, particularly those led and endorsed by more senior staff in the organisation, can help to challenge the culture and promote more creative approaches to flexible working and working across hierarchies (Hafford-Letchfield and Chick, 2006c).

Needless to say, it is very important that any discriminatory incidents are dealt with firmly and promptly and that discrimination in the workplace is tackled in a constructive way with recording and reporting of any incidents monitored and evaluated. Your organisation will have a grievance and harassment policy and procedure, with the option of monitoring. You should ensure that complaints and grievance procedures are known throughout the organisation to be effective and confidential. Conducting exit interviews with employees who are leaving the organisation, with a member of staff not responsible for managing that staff member, combined with regular staff experience surveys can also tell you a lot about staff experience in the workplace as part of your monitoring and evaluation process.

Establishing a positive and collaborative ethos as discussed in Chapter 3, where a dialogue within the team about diversity is not viewed as something to be dealt with by certain individuals or groups, can be achieved by supporting a process that makes individuals and groups think about how difference makes them practise – through discussion, debate, inquiry and reflection. According to Begum (2007), a recurring problem in promoting diversity is that of there being a culture of fear, intimidation, embarrassment and unease about addressing issues, because if someone shows signs of uncertainty or a lack of knowledge then they will be perceived as being politically incorrect or discriminatory. She recommends encouraging the development of networks for staff in minority groups which can also help to explore how particular strategic issues relating to promoting diversity are progressed, if these are given proper terms of reference and also networked into consultation structures with senior management. Translating recent legislation and guidance into practical, accessible and meaningful local policies can help support flexible working patterns that allow people to combine paid work with other responsibilities or aspirations. For example, this can combat the evidence that women with caring responsibilities tend to reduce their hours or work in areas that are less demanding than their qualifications or experience would suggest. According to Moriarty (2004), supporting carers in the workplace is not simply a question of altruism but is effective in terms of recruitment, retention and loss of productivity (this goes without saying where 70 per cent of couples with children were known to be working full time in 2000 (Bond et al., 2002)). Gender issues in combining family and work with equal rights in the workplace in order to reconcile the demands made by work and family life, given the number of women working in the social care workforce, speak for themselves. Actions such as implementing management training in family/carers policies, and selling the benefits for the organisation of introducing policies and practices which help employees obtain a better balance between their work and the rest of their lives, are likely to improve staff retention.

In relation to workforce planning, generating evidence from monitoring and evaluation to address any issues or gaps in workforce diversity should involve and engage staff. This can help them to appreciate and understand what their organisation is trying to achieve and the implications of what any data reveal. Similarly, if managers encourage staff to contribute to the evaluation of changes in policy and procedures or to develop new initiatives by drawing on their knowledge and expertise, which is similar to what we want to achieve with service users, then there is a greater chance that not only will evaluations be better informed. According to Begum there will be a greater degree of cooperation in implementing any changes (Begum, 2007).

Any workforce plans should have a clear commitment to the work-life balance in order to ensure its future. The DfEE (2000) offers the following checklist for employers, stating that an employer committed to work life balance

- recognises that effective practices to promote the work-life balance will benefit the organisation and its employees;

- acknowledges that individuals at all stages of their lives work best when they are able to achieve an appropriate balance between work and all other aspects of their lives;

- highlights the employer's and employee's joint responsibility to discuss joint solutions and encourages a partnership between individuals and their line manager;

- develops appropriate policies and practical responses that meet the specific needs of the organisation and its employees, having regard to fairness and consistency, valuing employees for their contribution to the business not for their work patterns, monitoring and evaluation;

- communicates their commitment to work-life strategies to its employees;

- demonstrates leadership from the top of the organisation and encourages managers to lead by example. **(DfEE, 2000, p4)**

As a manager, you may be in a position to advocate for staff at a more senior level for changes to work policies, procedures and practices that promote some of the above factors. At a local level you can make adjustments and develop a partnership approach with staff which maximises their contribution and recognises their potential.

C H A P T E R   S U M M A R Y

Challenges to the social care workforce have resulted in many new initiatives to try and overcome these. In this chapter we have looked at just a few of these by focusing on areas you may have more direct influence on or control over. All of the these are directly related to staff retention – an important aspect of any strategy in which managers can take an active role to promote. Strategies contributing towards retention include strengthening the quality and availability of workplace supervision; attention to the limits and boundaries of the social work role; flexibility in employment hours and patterns for those with difficulties in the workplace and a drive to increase awareness; and the rights and needs of employees with problems in the workplace (Stanley et al., 2007). Work in social care is both stressful and rewarding. If the social care sector cannot offer its members the support and structures they require to manage the demands of the work within the workplace, the outcome may be further isolation of staff from the communities that they serve and the quality of the services provided. The education and training of all social care practitioners should aim to promote their understanding of the proposed culture changes; person-centred working; empowering practice based on the social model; partnership working; and organisational learning at all levels (SCIE, 2005). According to research done by SCIE, ethical and empowering relationships between staff, service users and their carers are among the most essential vehicles for delivering support which is person-centred, proactive and seamless.

> *An appropriate workforce development strategy is not some 'add on' to the new vision but an integral element in its realisation. The vision will fail unless the workforce understands, owns and is properly equipped to deliver it. (SCIE, 2005)*

This begins with recruitment, where attracting staff from a diverse range of backgrounds committed to the values of social care is the first step to meeting the needs of service users and attaining outcomes. Thereafter the attention that managers give to workforce development through supervision, support and good role modelling is likely to instil in staff a greater sense of wellbeing and satisfaction about their work which will then in turn translate into greater productivity, improved performance and high quality services.

URTHER
EADING

Hawkins, P and Shohet, R, (2006) *Supervision in the helping professions.* Berkshire: McGraw-Hill and the Open University.
Provides a comprehensive account of developments and writing in the field of supervision across a number of professional disciplines.

Letchfield, T, Leonard, K, Begum, N and Chick, N F (2007) *Leadership and Management in Social Care.* London: Sage.
Written principally for leaders and managers of practice as well as other people responsible for staff development in social work and social care organisations, this book is not about management but examines the role and responsibilities that managers hold alongside other professionals for promoting and facilitating learning in the workplace, a role that is not always emphasised in traditional management texts.

Kirkton, G and Greene, AM (2000) *The Dynamics of Managing Diversity: a critical approach.* London: Butterworth-Heinemann.
Offers an integrative approach looking at all the issues surrounding managing equality and diversity

in the workplace. Equality and diversity are treated as mutually reinforcing rather than competitive concepts. The topics explored are firmly placed within the organisational and labour market framework and examined from a sociological perspective. The text draws on practical examples which have made a significant contribution to managing equality and diversity.

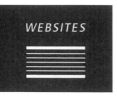

WEBSITES

www.cehr.org.uk *The Commission for Equality and Human Rights* was established in October 2007 by the Equality Act 2006 and is a non-departmental body and independent influential champion whose purpose is to reduce inequality, eliminate discrimination, strengthen good relations between people and protect human rights. The CEHR will bring together the work of the three existing Commissions, the Commission for Racial Equality (CRE), the Disability Rights Commission (DRC) and the Equal Opportunities Commission (EOC), in this new body and as one single source of information and advice will take on the powers of existing commissions, as well as new powers to enforce legislation more effectively and promote equality.

www.skillsforcare.org.uk *Skills for Care* is a national organisation working in consultation with carers, employers and service users to modernise adult social care in England, by ensuring qualifications and standards continually adapt to meet the changing needs of people who use care services. A number of policy documents and guidance on these can be obtained from the website particularly those relevant to workforce development issues.

www.cwdcouncil.org.uk *Children's Workforce Development Council* represents all children's services in workforce development issues, including Early Years, educational welfare, foster care and social care. It aims to improve outcomes for children and young people by enhancing the role of the workforce; to strengthen the workforce by ensuring that all workers have the appropriate skills and qualifications; to encourage integration while continuing to value the distinctiveness of each profession and to promote a vision of the children's workforce as integrated, satisfying and valuable.

Conclusion – twelve steps to designing your quality and performance management system

Assessing the quality of social care services and measuring their performance, either alongside or integrated within other public services such as health, housing and education, have become defining issues for all those involved. The way in which care and support services are being shaped and developed is beginning to rely on the use of information about quality and performance in a way that was inconceivable even just a decade ago. However, problems of eliciting reliable and useful information to evaluate what we do on a local basis remain. Some of these problems are at a conceptual level, concerning the question of what we are trying to evaluate; some attempt to find the right tools to measure or devise relevant data and analyse it effectively. Others are at a technical level, such as how we disseminate information about the quality and performance of the services we manage, particularly in a way which can be used by front-line staff to directly improve their work with users and carers (Challis et al., 2007, p2).

Throughout this book we have established that you will need to design and develop a system that is holistic and realistic in order to help to ensure that your organisation has the potential to deliver services that are high quality, achievable, cost-effective. As a concluding chapter, what follows is designed to briefly summarise some of the most important aspects of a quality assurance and performance monitoring systems, and to provide a quick reference guide or checklist for use in your local teams and service area.

The Department of Trade and Industry describes two basic approaches to quality management implementation. The first is a blitz approach where the whole organisation is exposed very rapidly to concepts, and mass education is started (p6). This can lead to many problems where people feel overwhelmed and confuses wholesale implementation with 'business as usual'. Ideologically, the lack of progress in social care around implementation is said to have gone hand-in-hand with a still-dominant concern that business ethics and principles are being used to control practitioners. This is said to be leading them away from a concern with the needs of service users towards a strategy that is more concerned with containing costs and ensuring accountability (Challis et al., 2007, p12). A second slower, planned, purposeful approach is therefore recommended, perhaps by implementing some of the ideas about good practice discussed in this book and where as a manager or practitioner you can have a small but steady influence. This is more likely to ensure that the core business of the organisation is simultaneous with the implementation of quality management systems in a near seamless transition. Hopefully, you did not find any of the topics in this book alien to your practice environment and that these reflected the underlying principles and practices of implementing issues being confronted. The following twelve steps should reinforce the quality issues in social work and social care;

1. Leadership for quality

We have seen, through the attention given to workforce development, that real improvement should come from the staff that we employ and the quality of the leadership they receive. An important first stage is for an organisation's leaders to be role models of a culture of quality of excellence so that these ideas permeate the organisation from the top. You can therefore think about your own leadership skills and the forums in which you may have some influence in order to introduce ideas on quality improvement and to get support for their implementation. Peters (1995) talks about the importance of managers keeping in touch with customers and people by *walking about* and using three major activities: listening – which suggests caring; teaching – in order to transmit values; and facilitating – by being able to give on-the-spot help. This can be a tough challenge for busy managers working within tight schedules, but combined with regular and detailed supervision can prevent any small problems from escalating later on.

2. Achieving a balance in assessing and measuring performance

Throughout this book we have looked at the different areas of a quality assurance framework, many of which were referred to in the Excellence model. Many issues have been identified; for example, the need to demonstrate service user involvement, to identify clear outcomes in consultation with users and carers, to establish realistic costings and to develop the ability to learn from best practice or research and evaluation. Kaplan and Norton's 'balanced scorecard' for public sector organisations (1996) measures an organisation's performance on five perspectives: the achievement of its strategic objectives; service users' and stakeholders' satisfaction; organisational excellence; taking account of financial targets; innovation and learning. We have managed to touch on many of these areas within the limitations of this book.

The main point being made here is that it is vital that, in improving overall performance, a framework is used that facilitates a balanced approach and accurately reflects and prioritises an organisation's most important areas. Some of these will inevitably be subject to constraints or be controversial, depending on whose perspective is being promoted. It is important, therefore, to open up and centre any ongoing debate on what exactly is being assessed and measured, and to keep this focused on the effective pursuit of service provision at the local level as well as the value of the procedures necessary to achieve this. Central government has an advantage through its performance measurement systems in being able to provide feedback on the bigger picture, but this information should be used to benefit local services generally rather than being used as a stick to beat them with.

3. Measure and monitor only what's important!

Front-line staff should be able to see the relationship between measured performance, good practice and good outcomes for service users. We have argued throughout this book that it is the role of both senior and front-line managers to ensure that all staff can reconcile these three. Involving service users and carers in establishing outcome measures should reflect what is important to them so that staff can involve them in developing action plans to make sure that services meet their needs. For example, users are usually left out of the process of devising performance indicators (Cutler and Waine, 1997). Data collection around case recording and activities involving these action plans can in turn be useful for performance measurement, but there should be no double entry of data to different systems.

This is one of the major challenges for managers when designing and implementing plans for improvements in order that these are understood up and down the line and that any performance indicators are relevant at a team level. Information should be made available to teams to ensure that they can manage their local performance responsibilities. A planning cycle and performance management process that incorporate front-line concerns and service users concerns, as well as government expectations, must have a better chance than something that feels imposed from above. This should take into account multi-disciplinary environment and stakeholder considerations, for example using different levels of aggregation within and across agencies to reflect patterns of variation which could merit further investigation and to more fully inform any differences in practice. As we saw in Chapter 5, engaging practitioners in enquiry as to the most effective modes of working and using practice wisdom, as well as more centrally-driven evidence, can be very effective and empowering.

4. Participatory approaches to development for quality

Measures that are seen by staff as irrelevant, unrealistic, inappropriate or unfair will be counterproductive (Moullin, 2004). If staff are involved in determining the measures and feel involved, they are likely to respond to those measures and to work with the management team in achieving them. Workforce development is very important and attention to good quality supervision and staff development can improve the recruitment and retention issues that have plagued social care organisations. We know for service users that consistency at first contact with them and the allocation of work at this point can influence their outcomes more positively. This could involve managing and monitoring initial referral systems, as well as giving attention to practical problem-solving in front-line services. Finding out why services deviate from planned targets, or whether these targets are achievable or justified, enables cases to be monitored with reference to key objectives. Challis et al. (2007, p249) cite the use of regular workshops in Cheshire which involved the participation of staff at all levels in the organisation, using a locally-based case review system to monitor and investigate performance.

5. Include both qualitative and quantitative performance indicators

It is important to have a balance between perception measures obtained directly from service users and other stakeholders and performance indicators which are recorded directly by an organisation. We have looked at different measurement tools in this book and drawn attention to the process of providing support as well as the potential outcomes. You should aim to use a combination of outcome and process measures, as both are important. Process measures, as we saw in the Excellence Model, are important because they measure the way in which the service is delivered which in turn is important to service users and carers. One of the difficulties with outcome measures is that these may be available only months or even years after the intervention or service has been delivered, by which time the people or service may have changed. However, there is also a danger in using process measures if these are not clearly linked to outcomes measures or service user satisfaction (Moullin, 2004). A service may then conform to process measures used but bear little relation to service users outcomes or satisfaction. Caution should be expressed in devising too many indicators as this will lead to information-overload and suspicion from those involved in the whole enterprise.

6. Be creative and stimulate innovation and learning

The only effective way of delivering service reform is by involving and stimulating the people who are going to deliver it. Staff need to be engaged in thinking how services can develop using their knowledge and experience. Organisations demonstrating service improvement are those that engage their front-line staff by listening to them, encouraging innovation and using their ingenuity, thus involving them in improvement and change (CSCI, 2007). Education and training are essential prerequisites for any organisation that learns. We have considered the usefulness of research and evidence in social care and the challenges in translating these into practices that practitioners can relate to and evaluate for themselves.

7. Use and exploit the potential of technology

The impact of new technologies in social care enters every aspect of an organisations' management and the delivery of services, as well as having a profound impact on the way we live and work. Social work is highly devoted to strong interpersonal relationships among all stakeholders and the role of technology is to support this aspect of professionalism and not to dominate it. Weiner and Petrella (2007) recommend two ways that social care managers can view the potential of electronic technologies. The first is their use for specific applications, the second to shape our lives and environment in more general ways (p221). Examples which they give of the former include the use of technology in dealing with the overwhelming amount of paperwork and record-keeping required for the continuous stream of transactions in social care. Technology can provide us with an analytical machine which enables us to pull data from a large number of sources and manipulate them in different ways to analyse and better understand social problems, for example, in analysing community demographics or the uptake of services. Electronic technology can serve as an information system for processing data which enable the development of care that can adapt to continuously changing environments.

Ensure that you and your staff are able to make the most of technologies by keeping your own skills and knowledge up to date in this area and by taking advantage of ITC training and any opportunities to be involved in the design of more user-friendly systems. The Web is also an important tool and resource for users, carers, employees and policy makers, and electronic communication can facilitate and support commu- nications between people and networking amongst different agencies and service providers. Technology has taken over a large amount of automaton-type processes in organisations, freeing up social care workers to undertake activities that only humans can perform. These are all issues that need to be recognised and understood in order to develop a balanced technology – use policy (Weiner and Petronella, 2007).

The use of technology to speed things up has to have a purpose, by improving opportunities for more personal and human interactions between people. Technol- ogy can improve the quality of services by enabling users to make appointments, get reminders, process payments, find information, use the 'chat room' facility to participate in mutual support groups and to undertake their own assessments fol- lowing the example given in Chapter 2 from West Sussex. There should be a continuous development of innovative uses of electronic technologies for care ser- vices that provide direct technology for users and staff. Managing information in a social work organisation has become as important as other management tasks. It does raise a number of legal and ethical issues around consent and confidentiality that need to be considered when pooling information, such as in the Identification, Referral and Tracking System for children's services. Any systems used to support service delivery can facilitate the notion of one virtual agency in which services are shaped and provided more holistically. Therefore, it is recommended that technol- ogies are used appropriately and thoughtfully to exploit their potential for strengthening all aspects and dimensions of social care services.

8. Achieving a balance between quality and costs

The number of performance measures used in social care and across the sector gen- erally looks set to increase. However, performance measures are useful only if their benefits outweigh the costs of obtaining them. Performance measurement is in itself part of how an organisation is managed and so it also needs to be cost effective and to deliver value. In foster care, for example, there are numerous standards for each looked-after child and it is clearly impossible for one organisation or social worker to monitor them all – this is where partnership working is important. It is better to have a smaller number of key measures that can be monitored and to integrate these with supervision and staff appraisal. Investing in prevention is a contentious and difficult area in social care which involves the capacity to evaluate local need, articulate a vision, and move resources towards this. The capacity to evaluate need is the building block to developing an effective, responsive, social care commissioning strategy. Com- missioning, as opposed to procurement and contracting strategies, should not simply be about finding services for those who need care, but should also be about devel- oping local services so that the right mix of services and facilities is available when these are needed.

9. Meet your strategic objectives through creative commissioning

Commissioning is at the heart of effective social care, offering an opportunity to transform people's lives through better services – which is not just about proce- dures and processes. *Every Child Matters* (DfES, 2003) and *Our health, or care, our say* (DoH, 2006a) both set out a clear vision for integrated services and make personalised care a priority. The Wanless review of social care for older people (Wanless, 2006) made clear that additional money should not be forthcoming without a commitment to reconfigure services. Taking a strategic long-term view of the sorts of services that need to be developed, based on the individual as well as the community, needs to involve finding better ways of listening to people, particularly those with complex needs who cannot participate in conventional consultations but who also have the right to live as independently as they can. Commissioners also need to engage with local economic development strategies to encourage the local market for care, recognising that the whole community must be served as well as those whose care needs to be funded. From 2007, effectiveness at strategic commissioning and purchasing became part of the annual performance assessment framework for councils (CSCI, 2006).

10. Avoid blame cultures and develop reward systems

Performance measurement systems should be focused on continuous improvement, i.e. ensuring that services are actually improved for service users and carers. It is easy when measures raise issues of concern, for these to be used to blame staff and thus contributing to a blame culture. In these situations, the emphasis needs to be on establishing what went wrong and how this issue can be addressed in the future, based on any learning. However, if management responds by blaming an individual or department, this will be counterproductive. One of the main problems with UK star rating systems is that there are penalties for organisations seen to be falling below the minimum requirements, and this can have implications for senior managers massaging information or achieving targets at the expense of real developments for service users and staff. Many debates on the development of and need for measuring quality and performance centre on their use in upholding or demonstrating accountability or making the activities of professionals and the processes within agencies more visible. According to Elcock (1983), there are many different strands to accountability. Accountability can be horizontal; across colleagues and managers, requiring that professionals adopt a clear monitoring process for their work, or vertical; up towards senior management and elected bodies, or downwards; to users and carers requiring that those with delegated authority are answerable for their actions. Challis et al. (2007) include budgetary, managerial, political and professional interpretations of what is meant by accountability – and as a manager, you will have to be sensitive to all of these dimensions.

There are a number of accreditation systems which organisations can incorporate to demonstrate their commitment to quality, such as Investors in People or Charter Marks. These can be useful in improving an organisation's image, and by making an explicit link between human resource practices and organisational performance in relation to recruitment and retention.

11. Translating feedback from performance measurement and quality assurance into a strategy for action and continuous improvement

With the current emphasis on collecting information in organisations and feeding this into monitoring and management structures, we do not always consider the importance of an effective system for translating this feedback into a more local strategy for action. The RADAR cycle (Results, Approach, Deploy, Assess and Review) used in the Excellence Model is an example of a systematic approach for translating feedback into action (www.dti.org.uk). In the results phase, measures are analysed comparing current with previous and desired performance. The next two phases identify the approaches needed to improve performance and deploy these throughout an organisation. The fourth phase is to assess and review the new approaches and the measures used, before starting the cycle again.

12. Recognising that quality assurance means change

In most social care organisations, quality assurance is still a new phenomenon. In essence this means the introduction of change where the theories and methods related to planned change are relevant. In planning a change strategy, you need to be familiar with the literature on organisational development systems analysis, adult learning and organisational sociology (Jessee, 1981, cited in Vuori, 2007). The key elements of planned change are the identification and demonstration of a need, an assessment of readiness and the capability to change, as well as a change strategy (Vuori, 2007). According to Vuori, things are not likely to change unless the current situation is perceived as unsatisfactory. Even a cursory look at existing routine statistics or collated performance indicators may arouse curiosity and can sometimes lead to questions about whether these are associated with the quality of care. To answer this question, more rigorous and time-consuming study may be needed to analyse the extent, nature and cause of the problem. Yet a quality assurance approach may provide a possible solution to the problem. A situational analysis combined with a readiness for change are also dependent on the health and socio-economic environment, as well as on the prevailing political climate. Vuori (2007) concludes that a pluralistic approach is essential which includes identifying the target group you wish to influence. This could include targeting decision-makers and identifying which individuals are most committed to improving the quality of care. You will need to identify who can be depended on for support and can follow changes through, or who might oppose change and the source of their opposition.

When promoting or selling a quality assurance approach to different target groups, you may need to highlight the various motives. Authorities and administrators are probably most interested in accountability and the wider social economic motives such as cost-containment; service users will concentrate on their experiences, safety and wellbeing; providers will be taken up with professional factors as well as altruistic motives. If you are considering implementing a quality assurance system or initiative, you may question where it is best to start. Beginning at the top with senior management may be appropriate, but this runs the risk of establishing a quality control system which people will resent rather than a quality assurance system that people will support. A pilot project may be an effective method using a targetable area of services. Vuori (1982) concludes that the development of quality assurance must follow a clearly expressed political will from which the research community can take the lead, can clarify the concept of quality and can identify factors influencing the quality of care services, developing methodologically-sound quality assurance methods. As we saw in Chapter 5, if practitioners themselves are responsible for implementing evaluation and evidence-based practice, their experiences gained in practice can be fed back into the decision-making process, research and education.

The future of performance management, assessment and inspection

The current government has a clear vision of revitalised and improved public services, designed around the needs of individuals, rooted in the values of the community, empowering people and offering choice (CSCI, 2007). These aim to transform the way in which we work and put the service user and carer at the centre of everything that we do. Politicians, commissioners, service providers, practitioners and regulators are all having to work together differently in the interests of service users – all of which requires new ways of working, new approaches, new attitudes, better integration and new structures, which makes for a challenging agenda. Changes in the way services are delivered bring with them changes in the way they are inspected and regulated. It has been envisaged that arrangements will enable the capacity to make independent judgements across services, using corporate assessment to aggregate outcomes without a separate social care judgement. Joint frameworks for inspecting services, involving a number of different inspectorate bodies, will bring together the inspection and regulation of the quality of adult's and children's services and will extend their role through Ofsted and OfCARE together with the Audit Commission.

Challenges will come with the transition of children to adult services, particularly where the latter have not developed at the same pace as children's services and do not offer the same level of continuous support to carry a child towards independence and into to adult life. Paying attention to issues arising from the collaboration between children's and adult's services, to ensure proper support for users going through transition and for young carers, is vital. Good services rely on the intelligent analysis of need, the pooling of resources where required and strong direction and leadership. Removing old boundaries invariably creates new boundaries. Making a difference for people is not about organisational change, but about how well people work together on the ground.

Good luck!

References

Adair, J (1983) *Effective leadership*. London: Pan.

Adams, R (2002) Quality assurance, in R Adams, L Dominelli and M Payne (eds), *Critical practice in social work*. Basingstoke: Palgrave.

Adams, L, Beadle-Brown, J and Mansell, J (2006) Individual planning: an exploration of the link between quality of plan and quality of life. *British Journal of Learning Disabilities*, 34, 68–76.

Ahearn, KK, Ferris, GR, Hochwater, WA, Douglas C and Ammeter, A (2004) Leader political skill and team performance. *Journal of Management*, 30 (3), 309–27.

Allan, D (2004) *The national evaluation of the Children's Fund: some recommendations for the commissioning and use of local evaluation*. NECE, available at www.ne-cf.org/core_files/lets%20fi nal%20draft202.doc

Appreciative Inquiry Commons (2007) Available at: appreciativeinquiry.case.edu Accessed March 2007.

Argyris, S (1993) *Knowledge for action, a guide to overcoming barriers to organizational change*. San Francisco, CA: Jossey Bass.

Arnstein, SR (1969) A ladder of citizen participation in the USA. *Journal of the American Institute of Planners*, 35 (4), 216–224.

Association of Directors of Social Services (ADSS) (2004) *Race equality through leadership in social care*. London: Association of Directors of Social Services with Social Care Institute for Excellence, Commission for Social Care Inspection and Race Equality Unit.

Association of Directors of Social Services (ADSS) (2005) *Independence, well-being and choice: the ADSS response to the Green Paper on adult social care*. Available at: www.adss.org.uk Accessed 21 August 2005.

Audit Commission (2002) *Recruitment and retention: a public service workforce for the twenty first century*. London: Audit Commission.

Axford, N, Little, N, Morpeth, L and Weyts, A (2005) Evaluating children's services: recent metho-dological developments. *British Journal of Social Work*, 35 (1), 73–88.

Balloch, S, Andrew, T, Ginn, T, McLean, J and Williams, J (1995) *Working in the social services*. London: National Institute Social Work Research Unit.

Barker, RA (1997) How can we train leaders if we do not know what leadership is? *Human Relations*, 50 (4), 343–62.

Barry, M and Hallet, C (eds) (1998) *Social exclusion and social work: issues of theory, policy and practice*. Dorset: Russell House.

Bass, BM (1990) *Bass and Stogdill's handbook of leadership: theory, research, and managerial applications*. 3rd edition. New York: Free Press.

Beck, U (1992) *Risk society*. London: Sage.

Begum, N (2006) Doing it for themselves: participation and black and minority ethnic service users. *Participation Report 14*. Race Equality Unit and Social Care Institute for Excellence. Bristol: Policy.

Begum, N (2007) Promoting diversity and equality through learning, in T Hafford-Letchfield, K Leonard, N Begum and NF Chick (2007) *Leadership and management in social care*. London: Sage.

Bell, L and Osborne, R (2005) To protect or not to protect? Complaining vulnerable adults? That is the challenge. *International Journal of Health Care Quality Assurance*, 18 (5), 385–394.

Benner, P (2001) *From novice to expert: excellence and power in clinical nursing practice*. Upper Saddle River, NJ: Prentice Hall/Pearson.

Bennett, P, Evans, R and Tattersal, A (1993) Stress and coping in social workers; a preliminary investigation. *British Journal of Social Work*, 23 (1), 31–44.

Beresford, P and Croft, S (1980) *Community control of social services departments*. London: Battersea Community Action.

Beresford, P and Croft, S (2001) Service users' knowledges and the social construction of social work. *Journal of Social Work*, 1 (3), 295–316.

Beresford, P and Croft, S (2004) Service users and practitioners reunited: the key component for social work reform. *British Journal of Social Work*, 34, 53–68.

Beresford, P, Adshead, L and Croft, S (2006) Service users' views of palliative care social work. *Findings*, November, Joseph Rowntree Trust.
Available at: www.jrf.org.uk/knowledge/findings/socialcare/1969.asp

Berman Brown, R and Bell, L (1998) Patient-centred audit: a user quality model. *Managing Service Quality*, 8 (2), 88–96.

Biestek, F (1961) *The casework relationship*. London: Allen and Unwin.

Boje, DM and Dennehey, R (1999) *Managing in the postmodern world*. Dubuque, IA: Kendall Hunt.

Bolton, M (2003) *Voluntary sector added value*. London: NCVO.

Bond, S, Hyman, J, Summers, J and Wise, S (2002) *Family friendly working? Putting policy into practice*. York: Joseph Rowntree Foundation.

Boud, D and Walker D (2002) Promoting reflection in professional courses, in R Harrison, A Hanson and J Clarke (eds). *Supporting lifelong learning, volume 1: perspectives on learning*. London: RoutledgeFalmer and the Open University.

Branfield, F, Beresford, P, Andrews, EJ, Chambers, P, Staddon, P, Wise, G and Williams-Findlay, B (2006) *Making user involvement work: supporting user networking and knowledge*. York: Joseph Rowntree Foundation. Available at www.jrf.org.uk

Brown, A (1998) *Organisational culture*. 2nd edition. London: Financial Times/Pitman.

Brown, HC (1998) *Social work and sexuality: working with lesbians and gay men*. London: Macmillan.

Bryans, P and Mavin, S (2003) Women learning to become managers: learning to fit in or to play a different game? *Management Learning*, 34 (1), 111–34.

Buono, AF, Bowditch, JL and Lewis, JW (1985) When cultures collide: the anatomy of a merger. *Human Relations*, 38 (5), 477–500.

Butt, J (2005) Are we there yet? Identifying the characteristics of social care organisations that successfully promote diversity in Butt, J, Patel, B and Stuart, O (eds) *Race equality discussion papers*. London: Social Care Institute for Excellence. Available in print and online at www.scie.org.uk

Butt, J and Davey, B (1997) The experience of black workers in the social care workforce, in M May, E Brundson and G Craig (eds), *Social Policy Review 9*, 141–61.

Buxton, V, James, T and Harding, W (1998) Using research in community nursing. *Nursing Times*, 94, (35) 2 September.

Cabinet Office, Performance and Innovation Unit (2004) *Strengthening leadership in the public sector*. Available from www.cabinetoffice.gov.uk

Cameron, KS and Quinn, E (1999) *Diagnosing and changing organisational culture: based on the competing values framework*. Massachusetts: Addison Wesley.

Cameron, A, Lart, R, Harrison, L, Macdonald, G and Smith, R (2000) *Factors promoting and obstacles hindering joint working: a systematic review*. Bristol: School for Policy Studies, Bristol University.

Carr, S (2004) *Has service user participation made a difference to social care services?* Position Paper no 3. London: Social Care Institute for Excellence. Available at: www.scie.org.uk

Challis, D, Clarkson, P and Warburton, R (2007) *Performance indicators in social care for older people*. Aldershot: Ashgate.

Challis, D, Darton R and Steart, K (1998) Linking community care and health care: a new role for secondary health care services, in D Challis, R Darton and K Stewart (eds), *Community care, secondary health care and care management*. Aldershot: Ashgate.

Charities Evaluation Service (2006) *Using an outcomes approach in the voluntary and community sector*. Charities Evaluation Services and the Public Interest and Non-profit Management research Unit, Open University Business School. Maidenhead: Open University.

Children and Young Persons' Unit (2001) *Learning to listen: core principles for the involvement of children and young people*. Nottinghamshire: DfES. Available at: www.dfes.gov.uk/cypu

Clarke, J (ed.) (1993) *A crisis in care: challenges to social work.* London: Sage.

Clegg, M (2002) Curriculum evaluation: is there an enlightened approach? UK Evaluation Society. www.evaluation.org.uk

Clegg, S, Kornberger, M and Pitsis, T (2005) *Managing and organisations: an introduction to theory and practice.* London: Sage.

Commission for Health Improvement (2002) *What is CHI?* London: CHI. www.chi.nhs.uk/eng/about.whatischi.shtml

Commission for Health Improvement (undated) *Sharing the learning on patient and public involvement from CHI's work: i2i – involvement to improvement*. London: CHI. Available at: www.chi.nhs.uk

Commission for Social Care Inspection (2005a) *Safeguarding children: the second joint chief inspectors' report on arrangements to safeguard children*. Crown copyright, produced by CSCI on behalf of the Joint Inspectorate Steering group. Available at: www.csci.org/uk/publications

Commission for Social Care Inspection (2005b) *The state of social care in England 2004–05.* Available at www.csci.org.uk/publications

Commission for Social Care Inspection (2005c) *Getting the best from complaints – the children's view: what children and young people think about the government's proposals to change the social services complaints procedures*. London: Commission for Social Care Inspection. Available at: www.csci.org.uk/publications/childrens_rights_director_reports/getting_the_best_from+_complaints_childrens_views.pdf

Commission for Social Care Inspection (2006) *Relentless optimism: creative commissioning for per-sonalised care, report of a seminar held by the Commission for Social Care Inspection on 18 May 2006.* Available from www.csci.org.uk/publications

Commission for Social Care Inspection (2007a) *Definitions – people who use services and experts by experience: guidance for staff.* Available at; www.csci.org.uk/get_involved/ Accessed 14 April 2007.

Commission for Social Care Inspection (2007b) *The future of performance management, assessment and inspection within children's services,* speech by Dame Denise Platt DBE, Chair, Commission for Social Care Inspection. Local government chronicle conference 'Policy changes in children's services', 28 February. Available at: www.cscie.org.uk

Commission for Social Care Inspection and National Statistics Office (2005) *Social services perfor-mance assessment framework indicators 2004–05.* Available at: www.csci.org.uk/publications

Community Care Needs Assessment Project (2007). *Asking the experts, a guide to involving people in shaping health and social care services.* Available at: www.ccnap.org.uk/guide/part1.htm Accessed 14 April 2007.

Cooper, A (2005) Surface and depth in the Victoria Climbié inquiry report. *Child and Family Social Work,* 10, 1–9.

Cooperrider, DL., Whitney, D and Stavros, JM, (2003) *Appreciative inquiry handbook: the first in a series of AI workbooks for leaders of change.* Ohio: Lakeside Communications.

Corby, B (2004) The costs and benefits of the North Wales Tribunal of Inquiry in N Stanley and J Manthorpe (eds), *The age of the inquiry: learning and blaming in health and social care.* London and New York: Routledge.

Corrigan, P and Leonard, P (1978) *Social work practice under capitalism, a Marxist approach.* London: Macmillan.

Cowden, S and Singh, G (2007) The 'user': friend, foe or fetish?: A critical exploration of user involvement in health and social care. *Critical Social Policy,* 27, 5–23.

Crisp, BR, Anderson, M, Orme, J and Lister, PG (2003) *Learning and teaching in social work educa-tion: assessment knowledge review 1.* London: Social Care Institute for Excellence (SCIE).

Crother-Laurin, C (2006) Effective teams: a symptom of healthy leadership. *The Journal for Quality & Participation,* Fall, 5–8.

Cutler, T and Waine, B (1997) *Managing the welfare state: text and sourcebook.* Oxford: Berg.

Dalrymple, J and Burke, B (2003) *Anti-oppressive practice, social care and the law.* Buckingham: Open University.

Davidson, MJ (1997) *The black and ethnic minority women manager: cracking the concrete ceiling.* London: Sage.

Davies, K and Hinton, P (1993) Managing quality in local government and the health service. *Public Money and Management,* 51.

Davis, SM (1984) *Managing corporate culture.* Cambridge: Ballinger.

de Bruijn, H (2001) *Managing performance in the public sector.* London and New York: Routledge.

Department for Education and Employment (DfEE) (2000) *Changing patterns in a changing world: a discussion document.* London: DfEE.

Department for Education and Skills (DfES) (2003) *Every Child Matters*. London: The Stationery Office.

Department for Education and Skills (DfES) (2004) *Working together: giving children and young people a say.* London: DfES. Available at: publications.teachernet.gov.uk/eOrderingDownload/DfES-0134-2004.doc

Department for Education and Skills (DfES) (2005a) *Championing children: a shared set of skills, knowledge and behaviours for those leading and managing integrated children's services* (draft). Nottingham: DfES.

Department for Education and Skills (DfES) (2005b) *Multi-agency working: toolkit for managers of multi-agency teams*. London: The Stationery Office.

Department for Education and Skills and Department of Health (DfES/DoH) (2006) *Options for excellence: building the social care workforce of the future*. Available at: www.dfes.gov.uk

Department of Environment, Transport and the Regions (DETR) (1998) *Modernising local government: improving local services through best value*. London: DETR.

Department of Health (DoH) (1989) *Caring for people: community care in the next decade and beyond*. London: HMSO.

Department of Health (DoH) (1997) *Shaping Our Lives*. London: The Stationery Office.

Department of Health (DoH) (1998) *Modernising social services, promoting independence, improving protection, raising standards* (CM4169). London: The Stationery Office.

Department of Health (DoH) (1999a) *National service framework for mental health: modern standards and service models.* London: The Stationery Office.

Department of Health (DoH) (1999b) *The government's objectives for children's social services (Quality Protects).* London: The Stationery Office.

Department of Health (DoH) (2000a) *A quality strategy for social care*. London: DoH.

Department of Health (2000b) *Shifting the balance of power within the NHS: securing delivery*. London: DoH.

Department of Health (DoH) (2000c) *The NHS: A plan for investment, a plan for reform*. London: DoH.

Department of Health (DoH) (2000d) *Framework for the assessment of children in need and their families*. London: DoH.

Department of Health (DoH) (2001a) *National minimum standards: care homes for older people.* London: The Stationery Office.

Department of Health (2001b) *Valuing people: a new strategy for learning disability for the 21st century*. London: The Stationery Office.

Department of Health (DoH) (2001c) *National service framework for older people.* London: DoH.

Department of Health (DoH) (2005a) *Building and nurturing an improvement culture. Improvement Leaders' Guides no 3*. London: DoH. Also available at www.modern.nhs.uk/improvementguides

Department of Health (DoH) (2005b) *Leading improvement: Improvement Leaders' Guides no 6*. London: DoH. Also available at: www.modern.nhs.uk/improvementguides

Department of Health (DoH) (2005c) *Research governance framework for health and social care*. Available at: www.dh.gov.uk/publications/guidance

Department of Health (DoH) (2005d) *Independence, wellbeing and choice: The vision for the future of social care in England*. A Green Paper. London: DoH.

Department of Health (DoH) (2006a) *Our health, our care, our say*. London: The Stationery Office.

Department of Health (DoH) (2006b) *Reward and recognition, the principles and practice of service user payment and reimbursement in health and social care*. Available at: www.dh.gov.uk/en/Publicationsandstatistics/Publications/PublicationsPolicyAndGuidance/ DH_4138523 Accessed 14 April 2007.

Department of Health (DoH) (2006c) *Outcome-based commissioning*. Written notes from the commissioning e-book podcast, Care Services Improvement Partnership, pp 1–10. Available at: www.cat.csip.org.uk/commissioningebook

Department of Health (DoH) *Policy research programme: policy, aims and priorities*. Available at: www.dh.gov.uk/en/Policyandguidance/Researchanddevelopment/Policyresearchprogramme/DH 40001718

Department of Health and NHS Service Delivery and Organisation Research and Development Programme (2006) *New governance, more incentives: but can they really improve care?* Studying health care organisations, briefing paper, November. Available at: www.sdo.lshtm.ac.uk

Department of Trade and Industry (DTI) (undated) *The original quality gurus*. Available at: www.dti/ qualitygurus.gov.uk

Dominelli, L (1988) *Anti-racist social work*. Basingstoke: Macmillan.

Dominelli, L (1989) *Feminist social work*. Basingstoke: Macmillan.

Dominelli, L (1997) Feminist theory in Davies, M (ed.), *The Blackwell companion to social work*. Oxford: Blackwell.

Dominelli, L (2002) *Anti-oppressive social work theory and practice*. Basingstoke: Palgrave, Macmillan.

Donabedian, A (1969) *Medical care appraisal – quality and utilization. A guide on medical care administration*. American Public Health Association.

Donabedian, A (1980) *The definitions of quality and approaches to its assessment, vol. 1*. Michigan: Health Administration Press.

Donzelot, J (1988) *The policing of families: welfare versus the state*. London: Hutchinson.

Drummond, F, Torrance, GW, O'Brien, BJ and Sculpher, M (2005) *Methods for the evaluation of health care programmes*. Oxford: Oxford University Press.

Eborall, C (2003) *The state of the social care workforce in England: The first annual report of the Topss England Workforce Intelligence Unit*. Leeds: Topss England.

Eddy, DM (1992) *Assessing health practices and designing practice policies: the explicit approach*. Philadelphia: American College of Physicians.

Elcock, H (1983) *Policy and management in local authorities*. 3rd edition. London: Routledge.

Equal Opportunities Commission (2002) *Women and men in Great Britain: management*. Available at: www.eoc.org.uk Accessed 8 August 2006.

Equal Opportunities Commission (2003*) Facts about women and men in Great Britain*: annual compilation of gender statistics. London: EOC. Available at: www.eoc.org.uk

Eraut, M (2006) Editorial: learning contexts. *Learning in Health and Social Care*, 5 (1), 1–8.

Felton, K (2005) Meaning-based quality-of-life measurement: a way forward in conceptualising and measuring client outcomes? *British Journal of Social Work*, 35, 221–36.

Ferlie, E, and Steane, P (2002) Changing developments in NPM. *International Journal of Public Administration*, 25 (12), 1459–69.

Foster, P and Wilding, P (2000) Whither welfare professionalism? in J Reynolds, J Henderson, J Seden, J Charlesworth and A Bullman (eds) (2002) *The managing care reader*. London: Routledge/ Open University Press.

Francis, J and Netten, A (2004) Raising the quality of home care: a study of service users' views. *Social Policy and Administration*, 38 (3), 290–305.

Friday, E and Friday, SS (2003) Managing diversity using a strategic planned change approach. *Journal of Management Development*, 22, 863–80.

Gardner, JW (1990) *On leadership*. New York: Free Press.

Gastor, L (1995a) *Management skills in decentralise environments*. Luton: Local Government Management Board.

Gastor, L (1995b) *Quality in public services*. Buckingham: Open University.

Gatehouse, M and Ward, H (2003) *The use of informtion and information systems in local authority children's services. Final report on the data analysis network to the Wales Assembly Government.* Loughborough: Centre for Child and Family Research, University of Loughborough.

Gavin, DA (1984) What does product quality really mean? *Sloan Management Review*, 26, 25–43.

General Social Care Council (GSCC) (2005) *Post-qualifying framework for social work education and training*. London: GSCC.

General Social Care Council and King's College London (2006*) Diversity and progression in social work education in England: A report on progression rates among DipSW students*. London: GSCC and King's College.

Gerada, C and Cullen, R (2004) Clinical governance leads: roles and responsibilities. *Quality in Primary Care*, 12, 13–18.

Gilbert, M and Evans, K (2000) *Psychotherapy supervision in context: an integrative approach*. Buckingham: Open University.

Giovannini, M (2004) What gets measured gets done. *The Journal for Quality and Participation*, Winter, 21–6.

Glasby, J and Beresford, P (2006) Commentary and issues: who knows best? Evidence based practice and the service user contribution. *Critical Social Policy*, 26 (1), 268–84.

Godfrey, C (2001) Economic evaluation in health perspective in I Ruutman, M Goodstradt, B Hyndman, DV McQueen, L Potvin, J Springett and E Ziglio (eds) *Evaluation in Health Promotion: principles and perspectives*. Copenhagen: WHO Europe.

Goldberg, EM and Connolly, N (1982) *The effectiveness of social care for the elderly.* London: Heineman.

Goleman, D (1996) *Emotional intelligence: why it can matter more than IQ*. London: Bloomsbury.

Goleman, D (1998) *Working with emotional intelligence*. London: Bloomsbury.

Gordon, GG (1991) Industry determinants of organisational culture. *Academy of Management Review*, 16, 396–415.

Gould, N (2000) Becoming a learning organisation: a social work example. *Social Work Education*, 19 (6), 585–96.

Gray, A (2005a) Critical appraisal of methods: economic evaluation, in M Dawes, P Davies, A Gray, J Mant, K Seers and R Snowball (eds) *Evidence-based practice: a primer for health care professionals*. London, New York: Churchill Livingstone.

Gray, A (2005b) Is the intervention cost effective? in Dawes, M, Davies, P, Gray, A, Mant, J, Seers, K and Snowball, R (eds) *Evidence-based practice: a primer for health care professionals*. London, New York: Churchill Livingstone.

Green, J and South, J (2006) *Evaluation*. Berkshire, NY: Open University Press and McGraw-Hill Education.

Gregory, M and Holloway, M (2005) Language and the shaping of social work. *British Journal of Social Work*, 35, 37–53.

The Guardian (2006) 'Painfully slow' progress means women could take 200 years to win political equality. 5 February.

The Guardian (2007) The children's champions. *Society Guardian*, 28 February.

Habermas, J (1978) *Knowledge and human interests*. London: Heineman.

Hafford-Letchfield, T (2006a) *Management and organisations in social work*. Exeter: Learning Matters.

Hafford-Letchfield, T (2006b) Cultural revolution. Management in practice. *Community Care Magazine*, 3–9 August.

Hafford-Letchfield, T and Chick, NF (2006) Succession planning: developing management potential in a local authority social services department. *Diversity in Health and Social Care*, 3 (3), 193–201.

Hafford-Letchfield, T, Leonard, K, Begum, N and Chick, NF (2007) *Leadership and management in social care*. London: Sage.

Hammond, S (1998) *The thin book of appreciative inquiry*. Available from: info@thinbook.com

Handy, C (1995) *Gods of management: the changing work of organisations*. London: Arrow.

Harding, T (1997) *A life worth living: the independence and inclusion of older people*. London: Help the Aged.

Harlow, E (2004) Why don't women want to be social workers anymore? New managerialism, post feminism and the shortage of social workers in social services departments in England and Wales. *European Journal of Social Work*, 7, 167–79.

Harris, J (2003) *The social work business*. London: Routledge.

Harris, N (1987) Defensive social work. *British Journal of Social Work*, 17 (1), 61–9.

Harrison, R (2004) *Learning and development*. 4th edition. London: Chartered Institute of Personnel and Development.

Harrison, R and Stokes, H (1992) *Diagnosing organizational culture*. San Francisco; Pfeiffer/Jossey-Bass.

Hawkins, P and Shohet, R (2006) *Supervision in the helping professions*. 3rd edition. Berkshire: Open University Press and McGraw-Hill Education.

Healey, K (2002) Managing human services in a market environment: what role for social workers? *British Journal of Social Work*, 32, 57–74.

Health Care Commission, Commission for Social Care Inspection and Audit Commission (2005) *A review of progress against the National Service Framework for Older People*. Available at: www.csci.org.uk

Heffernan, K (2006) Social work, new public management and the language of 'service user'. *British Journal of Social Work*, 36, 139–47.

Henderson, J and Seden, J (2004) What do we want from social care managers? in Dent, M, Chandler, J and Barry, J (eds) *Questioning the new public management*. Aldershot: Ashgate.

Henkel, M (1991) *Government, evaluation and change.* London: Jessica Kingsley.

Henwood, M and Waddington, E (1998) *Listening to users of domiciliary care services: developing and monitoring quality standards.* Leeds: Nuffield Institute for Health.

Higgs, M (2003) How can we make sense of leadership in the 21st century? *Leadership & Organization Development Journal,* 24 (2), 116–31.

HMSO (1974) *Committee of enquiry into the care and supervision provided in relation to Maria Colwell.* London: HMSO.

Holloway, J (2001) *Understanding evaluation* (Block 1, no 18). Prepared for an Open University Business School course. Milton Keynes: Open University Press.

Horner, N (2003) *What is social work: context and perspectives.* Exeter: Learning Matters. Available at: www.learningmatters.co.uk

House, RJ (1995) Leadership in the twenty-first century in Howard, A (ed.) *The changing nature of work.* San Francisco, CA: Jossey-Bass.

Hudson, B (2005) "Not a cigarette paper between us": integrated inspection of children's services in England. *Social Policy and Administration*, 39 (5), 513–22.

Hughes, M, Traynor, T (2000) *Reconciling process and outcomes in evaluation*. 6(1) pp37–49.

Humphries, B (2004) An unacceptable role for social work: implementing immigration policy. *British Journal of Social Work*, 34, 93–107.

Huntington, J (1981) *Social work and general medical practice: collaboration or conflict?* London: Allen and Unwin.

Improvement and Development Agency (IDeA) (2004) *Prospects*. Study co-funded by Leadership Research and Development Ltd. Available at www.IDeA.org. uk

Jacobs, S and Rummery, K (2002) Nursing homes in England and their capacity to provide rehabilitation and intermediate care services. *Social Policy and Adminstration*, 26 (7), 735–52.

Jessee, WF (1981) Approaches to improving the quality of healthcare: organisational change. *Quality Review Bulletin* (July).

Johns, N and Jordan, B (2006) Social work, merit and ethnic diversity. *British Journal of Social Work*, 36(8), 1271–88.

Johnson, G (1989) Re-thinking incrementalism, in Asch, D and Bowman, C (eds) *Readings in strategic management*. London: Macmillan.

Jones, C (2001) Voices from the front line; state social workers and new labour. *British Journal of Social Work*, 31 (4), 547–62.

Jordan, B and Jordan, C (2000) *Social work and the third way: tough love as social policy*. London: Sage.

Kaplan, RS and Norton, DP (1996) *The balanced scorecard: translating strategy into action*. Harvard: Harvard Business School Press.

Kearney, P (2004) First line managers, the mediators of standards and the quality of practice in Statham, D (ed.) *Managing front line practice in social care*. (Research Highlights in Social Work 40) London: Jessica Kingsley.

King's Fund (1990) *The work of the Equal Opportunities Task Force 1986–1990: A final report*. London: King Edward's Hospital Fund for London.

King's Fund (1992) *Living options in practice, achieving user participation: planning services for people with severe physical and sensory disabilities* (Project Paper No 3). London: Kings Fund Centre.

Kitson, A, Harvey, G and McCormack, B (1998) Enabling the implementation of evidence based practice: a conceptual framework. *Quality in Health Care*, 7, 149–58.

Kotecha, N, Fowler, C, Donskoy, A, Johnson, P, Shaw, T and Doherty, K (2007) *A guide to user-focused monitoring, setting up and running a project*. London: Sainsbury Centre for Mental Health. Available at: www.scmh.org.uk

Kotter, JP (1990) *Forces for change: how leadership differs from management*. New York: Free.

Kotterman, J (2006) Leadership versus management: what's the difference? *The Journal for Quality & Participation*, Summer. Available at: www.asq.org

Laming, H (2003) *The Victoria Climbié Enquiry: report of an enquiry by Lord Laming*. London: DoH.

Lave, J and Wenger, E (2002) *Situated Learning: legitimate peripheral participation* (Learning in Doing: Social Cognitive and Computational Perspectives). Cambridge: Cambridge University Press.

Liff, S and Dale, K (1994) Formal opportunity, informal barriers: black women managers within a local authority. *Work, Employment and Society* 8 (2), 177–95.

Lindow, V (1999) Power, lies and injustice: the exclusion of service users voices in Parker, M (ed.) *Ethics and community in the health care profession*. London: Routeledge.

Lishman, J (2000) Evidence for practice: the contribution of research methodologies. Paper for Seminar 4 in the ERSC-funded *Theorising Social Work Series*. Cardiff, April.
Available at: www.nisw.org.uk/tswr/lishman.html/

Local Authority Workforce Intelligence Group (2006) *Adults, children and young people: local authority social care workforce survey, 2005*. (Report no 36, Social Care Workforce Series, July). Available at: www.lgar.local.gov.uk/lgv/aio/12503 Accessed 29 June 2007.

Lorbiecki, A (2001) Changing views on diversity management: the rise of the learning perspective and the need to recognize social and political contradictions. *Management Learning*, 32 (3), 345–61.

Lorenz, W (2006) Education for the social professions, in K Lyons and S Lawrence (eds) *Social work in Europe: educating for change.* London: Venture.

Lymbery, M (2001) Social work at the crossroads. *British Journal of Social Work*, 31(3), pp369–84.

Lymbery, M and Butler, S (eds) (2004) *Social work ideals and practical realities.* Basingstoke; Palgrave Macmillan.

Lyons, K and Lawrence, S (eds) (2006) *Social work in Europe: educating for change.* Birmingham: Venture.

Macdonald, G (2003) *Using systematic reviews to improve social care.* Bristol: The Policy Press for Social Care Institute for Excellence.

Malcolm, B (2007) Managing diversity in social services settings, in J Aldgate, L Healy, B Malcolm, B Pine, W Rose and J Seden (eds), *Enhancing social work management.* London, Philadelphia: Jessica Kingsley with the Open University.

Malin, N, Wilmot, S and Manthorpe, J (2002) *Key concepts and debates in health and social policy.* Buckinghamshire: Open University Press.

Marsh P and Fisher, M in collaboration with Mathers, N and Fish, S (2005) *Developing the evidence base for social work and social care practice.* (Using knowledge in social care, Report 10). Bristol: Policy Press, Social Care Institute for Excellence. Available at: www.scie.org.uk

Martin, V (2003) *Leading change in health and social care.* London: Routledge.

Martin, L and Kettner, P (1996) *Measuring the performance of human service programmes.* Thousand Oaks, CA: Sage.

Martin, V and Henderson, E (2001) *Managing in health and social care.* London: Routledge and the Open University Press.

McLean, J (2002) Commitment and work: social services employees. *MCC: Building Knowledge for Integrated Care*, 10 (4), 35–7.

McLean, J and Andrew, T (1998) *The Northern Ireland social services workforce: residential workers and qualifying training, a preliminary investigation into the careers of residential workers who become qualified.* London: National Institute for Social Work Research Unit.

McLenachan, J (2006) Facing up to a recruitment crisis. *The Guardian*, 27 November.

Means, R, Richards, S and Smith, R (2003) *Community care policy and practice.* 3rd edition. Basingstoke: Palgrave Macmillan.

Menzies, I (1970) *The functioning of social systems as a defence against anxiety.* London: Tavistock Institute of Human Relations.

Mitchell, W and Sloper, P (2003) Quality indicators: disabled children's and parents' prioritisations and experiences of quality criteria when using different types of support services. *British Journal of Social Work*, 33, 1063–80.

Moriarty, J (2004) *Main messages and bibliography from the NISW workforce studies* (Social care workforce intelligence unit). London: King's College, 2003.

Morrison, T (2002) *Staff supervision in social care: making a real difference for staff and service users.* Brighton: Pavilion.

Morrison, T (2007) Emotional intelligence, emotion and social work: context, characteristics, complications and contribution. *British Journal of Social Work*, 37, 245–63.

Moullin, M (2003) *Delivering excellence in health and social care.* Maidenhead: Open University Press.

Moullin, M (2004) Eight essentials of performance measurement (Guest editorial). *International Journal of Health Care Quality Assurance,* 17 (3), 110–12.

Munroe, E (2004) The impact of audit on social work practice. *British Journal of Social Work,* 34, 1075–95.

National Institute for Social Work Research Unit (NISW) (2000) *Research towards a human resource policy for social care.* London: National Institute for Social Work.

Nebecker, DM and Tatum, B C (2002) Understanding organisational processes and performance, in Lowman, RL (ed.), *Handbook of organizational consulting psychology.* San Francisco: Jossey-Bass, 668–91.

Normann, R (1978) *Development strategies for Swedish knowledge* (in Swedish). Stockholm: SIAR.

Ofsted (2004) *Every Child Matters: inspecting services for children and young people, discussion with stakeholders: summary of responses.* London: Ofsted.

Oliver, M (1996) *Understanding disability: from theory to practice.* Basingstoke: Macmillan.

Osmond, J and O'Connor, I (2004) Formalizing the unformalized: practitioners' communication of knowledge in practice. *British Journal of Social Work,* 34, 677–92.

PACE – Project for Advocacy, Counselling, and Education (2006). Available at: www.pace.org.uk Accessed18 April 2006.

Panskepp, J (2000) Emotions as natural kinds within the mammalian brain in Leis, M and Haviland-Jones, J (eds) *Handbook of emotions.* London: Guilford.

Parsloe, P and Stevenson, O (1978) *Social services teams.* London: HMSO.

Parton, N (1985) *The politics of child abuse.* Basingstoke: Macmillan.

Parton, N (2000) Some thoughts on the relationship between theory and practice in and for social work. *British Journal of Social Work,* 39, 449–63.

Patel, A (1994) Quality assurance (BS5750) in social services departments. *International Journal of Public Sector Management,* 7 (2), 4–15.

Patmore, C (2001) Can managers research their own services? An experiment in consulting frail, older community care clients. *Managing Community Care,* 9 (5), 8–17.

Patton, M (1997) *Utilization-focused evaluation.* 3rd edition. Thousand Oaks, CA: Sage.

Pawson, R, Boaz, A, Grayson, L, Long, A and Barnes, C (2003) Types and quality of knowledge in social care. *Knowledge Review No 3.* Bristol: Social Care Institute for Excellence with the Policy Press.

Paxton, W and Pearce (2005) *The voluntary sector delivering public services, transfer or transformation?* (Study papers: Part I). London: Joseph Rowntree Foundation.

Paxton, R, Whitty, P, Zaatar, Z, Fairbairn, A and Lothian, J (2006) Research, audit and quality improvement. *International Journal of Health Care Quality Assurance,* 19 (1), 105–11

Pelmutter, FD, Bailey, D and Netting, FE (2001) *Managing human resources in the human services: supervising challenges.* New York: Oxford University Press.

Percy-Smith, J (2002) *Promoting change through research: the impact of research on local government.* London: Joseph Rowntree Foundation.

Peters, T (1995) *The pursuit of WOW! Every person's guide to topsy-turvy times.* London: Macmillan.

Pfeffer, N and Coote, A (1991) *Is quality good for you? A critical review of quality assurance in welfare services* (Social Policy Paper No 5). London: Institute for Public Policy Research.

Pine, BA and Healy, LM (2007) New leadership for the human services: involving and empowering staff through participatory management in J Aldgate, L Healy, B Malcolm, B Pine, W Rose and J Seden, *Enhancing social work management; theory and best practice from the UK and USA.* London, Philadelphia: Jessica Kingsley.

Pinnock, M and Dimmock, B (2003) Managing for outcomes, in Henderson, J and Atkinson D (eds), *Managing care in context.* London, New York: Routledge.

Polanyi, M (1983) *The tacit dimension.* Gloucester, MA: Peter Smith.

Pollitt, C (2003) *The essential public manager.* London:McGraw-Hill International.

Pugh, R (1996) *Effective language in health and social work.* London: Chapman and Hall.

Qureshi, H, Patmore, C, Nicholas, E and Bamford, C (1998) *Overview: outcomes of social care for older people and carers* (Outcomes in Community Care Practice Series, No. 5). York: Social Policy Research Unit.

Qureshi, H and Henwood, M (2000) *Older people's definitions of quality services.* London: Joseph Rowntree Foundation.

Reid, Y, Johnson, S, Morant, N, Kuipers, E, Szmukler, E, Thornicroft, G, Bebbington, P and Prosser, D (1999) Explanations for stress and satisfaction in mental health professionals: a qualitative study. *Social Psychiatry and Psychiatric Epidemiology,* 34 (6), 310–18.

Research in Practice (2003) A review of literature on leading evidence informed practice (EIP). Available at: www.rip.org.uk

Ring, C (2001) Quality assurance in mental health-care: a case study from social work. *Health and Social Care in the Community*, 9 (6), 383–90.

Robinson, J and Banks, P (2005) *The business of caring: King's Fund inquiry into care services for older people in London.* London: King's Fund Publications.

Rudkin, A and Rowe, D (1999) A systematic review of the evidence base for lifestyle planning in adults with learning disabilities: implications for other disabled populations. *Clinical Rehabilitation*, 13, 362–72.

Sackett, DL (1987) Screening in family practice: prevention, levels of evidence, and the pitfalls of common sense. *Journal of Family Practice*, 24(3), 233–4.

Sackett, D, Rosenberg, W, Gray, J, Haynes, R and Richardson, W (1996) Evidence-based medicine: what it is and what it isn't. *British Medical Journal*, 312 (7023) 71–2.

Sale, DNT (2000) *Quality assurance: a pathway to excellence.* Basingstoke: Macmillan.

Sandars, J (2004) Knowledge management: something old, something new! *Work Based Learning in Primary Care,* 2, 9–17.

Schein, EG (1992) *Organisational culture and leadership.* 2nd edition. San Francisco, CA: Jossey-Bass.

Schmadl, JC (1979) Quality assurance: examination of the concept. *Nursing Outlook*, 27 (7), 462–5.

Schon, D (1991) *The reflective practitioner.* 2nd edition. Aldershot: Arena.

Schraeder, M, Tears, RS and Jordan, MH (2004) Organisational culture in public sector organisations: promoting change through training and leading by example. *Leadership and Organization Development Journal,* 26 (6), 492–502.

SCIE (2004) *Learning organisations: a self-assessment resource pack.* London: Social Care Institute for Excellence. Available in print or downloadable from www.scie.org.uk

SCIE (2005) *SCIE consultation response to independence, well-being and choice.* Available at: www.scie.org.uk

Scott, T, Mannion, R, Davies, TO and Marshall, MN (2003) Implementing culture change in health care: theory and practice. *International Journal for Quality in Health Care,* 15 (2), 111–18.

Scottish Workforce Unit (2006) *A toolkit for voluntary sector social services in Scotland.* (Toolkit co-ordinated by Caroline Sturgeon and Janet Miller.) Available at: www.ccpscotland.org/workforceunit/info/documents/WorkforcePlanningToolkit.pdf Accessed 3 April 2007.

Senge, P (1990) *The fifth discipline.* New York: Currency/Doubleday.

Shaping our Lives (1997) *Interim Report.* London: National Institute for Social Work.

Shaw, I (2004) *Evidence based social work practice: a review of developments.* Unpublished conference paper presented at the Inter-Centre Network for the Evaluation of Social Work Practice (Intsoceval), 7th annual workshop, 30 September–2 October, at the University of Applied Sciences, Slothurn, Switzerland.

Shaw, I (2005) Practitioner research: evidence or critique? *British Journal of Social Work,* 35, 1231–48.

Shaw, I, Greene, J and Mark, M (2006) *Handbook of evaluation: policy, programme and practice.* London: Sage.

Sheldon, B and Chilvers, R (2000) *Evidenced-based social care: a study of prospects and problems.* Lyme Regis: Russell House Publishing.

Sheppard, M (1995) Social work, social science and practice wisdom. *British Journal of Social Work,* 25, 265–93.

Sheppard, M, Newstead, S, Di Caccavo, A and Ryan, K (2000) Reflexivity and process knowledge in social work. *British Journal of Social Work,* 30 (4) 465–88.

Siebert, DC (2004) Depression in North Carolina social workers: implications for practice and research. *Social Work Research,* 28 (1), 30–40.

Simon, K (1995) Views from another angle: the professional perspective, in *"I'm not complaining but...".* London: Joseph Rowntree Trust. Available at: www.jrt.org.uk

Singh, V (2002) *Managing diversity for strategic advantage.* Available at: www.managementandleadershipcouncil.org.uk/reports/other.htm (Accessed 9 August 2006).

Skills for Care (2004a) *Leadership and management: a strategy for the social care workforce.* Available at: www.skillsforcare.org.uk

Skills for Care (2004b) *What leaders and managers in social care do – a statement for a leadership and management development strategy for social care* (No 1). Available at: www.skillsforcare.org.uk

Skills for Care (2004b) *Leadership and management 2006 update pack.* Available from: www.skillsforcare.org.uk

Smith, R (1992) Audit and research. *British Medical Journal*, 305 (6859), 905–6

Stanley, N, Manthorpe, J and White, W (2007) Depression in the profession: social workers' experiences and perceptions. *British Journal of Social Work*, 37, 281–98.

Steiner, A (2001) Intermediate care – a good thing? *Age and Ageing*, 30–S3: 33–9.

Stevenson, O (1998) *Child welfare in the UK*. Oxford: Blackwell Science.

Stevenson, O (2005) Genericism and specialization: the story since 1970. *British Journal of Social Work*, 35, 569–86.

Stone, AG, Russell, RF and Patterson, K (2004) Transformational versus servant leadership: a difference in leader focus. *Leadership and Organizational Development*, 25, 349–61.

Talwar, R (1993) – Available at www.dti.gov.uk/qualitytqm

Taylor, C and White, S (2006) Knowledge and reasoning in social work: educating for humane judgement. *British Journal of Social Work*, 36, 937–54.

Taylor, G. (1993) Challenges from the margin, in M Lymbery (2001) Social work at the crossroads. *British Journal of Social Work*, 31(3), pp 369-84.

Thompson, N, (2003) *Promoting equality: challenging discrimination and oppression*. 2nd edition. Basingstoke: Palgrave Macmillan.

Thyer, BA (2001) Evidence-based approaches to community practice in Briggs, HE and Corcoran, K (eds) *Social work practice: treating common client problems*. Chicago: Lyceum.

Tilbury, C (2004) The influence of performance measurement on child welfare policy and practice. *British Journal of Social Work*, 34, 225-41.

Tones, K and Tilford, S (2001) *Health promotion: effectiveness, efficiency and equity*. 3rd edition. Cheltenham: Nelson Thornes.

Townend, M (2005) Interprofessional supervision from the perspectives of both mental health nurses and other professionals in the field of cognitive behavioural psychotherapy. *Journal of Psychiatric and Mental Health Nursing*, 12, 582–88.

Training Organisation for Personal Social Services (TOPPS) (2000) *Modernising the social care workship: the first national training strategy for England*. Available from: www.topps.org.uk

Trice, HM and Beyer, JM (1993) *The cultures of work organisations.* Englewood Cliffs, NJ: Prentice-Hall.

Trivedi, P (2002) Let the tiger roar. *Mental Health Today* (August), 30–33.

Turner, M and Beresford, P (2005) *Contributing on equal terms. Service user involvement and the benefits system*. Bristol: Policy.

Tyson, K (1995) *New foundations for scientific social and behavioural research: the hereurisic paradigm.* Englewood Cliffs: Prentice-Hall.

Vuori, H (1982) *Patient satisfaction: an attribute or indicator of quality care?* Geneva: WHO.

Vuori, H (2007) Introducing quality assurance: an exercise in audacity. *International Journal of Health Care Quality Assurance*, 20 (1), 10–15.

Walker, P (2002) Understanding accountability: theoretical models and their implications for social services organisations. *Social Policy and Administration*, 36, 62–75.

Walker, S, Murray, B and Atkinson, D (2003) Quality matters, in J Henderson and D Atkinson (eds), *Managing care in context*. London, New York: Routledge and the Open University.

Walton, R (2005) Social work as a social institution. *British Journal of Social Work*, 35, 587–607.

Wanless, D (2006) *Securing good care for older people*. London: King's Fund Centre.

Ward, H (2004) Working with managers to improve services: changes in the role of research in social care. *Child and Family Social Work*, 9 (1), 13–25.

Watson, D (2004) Managing quality enhancement in the personal social services: a front-line assessment of its impact on service provision with residential childcare. *The International Journal of Public Sector Management*, 17 (2), 153–65.

Webb, SA (2006) Social work in a risk society: social and political perspectives. Basingstoke, New York: Palgrave Macmillan.

Weinberg, A, Williamson, J, Challis D and Hughes, J (2003) What do care managers do? A study of working practice in older people's services. *British Journal of Social Work*, 33, 901–19.

Weiner, ME and Petrella, P (2007) The impact of new technology: implications for social work and social care managers, in J Aldgate, L Healy, B Malcolm, B Pine, W Rose and J Seden (eds), *Enhancing social work management*. London, Philadelphia: Jessica Kingsley with the Open University.

Weinstein, J (2006) Involving mental health service users in quality assurance. *Health Expectations,* 9, 98–109.

Wenger, E (1998) *Communities of practice*. Cambridge: Cambridge University Press.

White, S and Stancombe, J (2003) *Clinical judgement in the health and welfare professions: extending the evidence base.* Maidenhead: Open University.

Williamson, JW (1979) Formulating priorities for quality assurance activity: descriptions of a method and its application. *Journal of the American Medical Association*, 329, 631–7.

Wilson, E (1975) *Women and the welfare state*. London: Tavistock.

Wright, F (2005) Lay assessors and care home inspections: is there a future? *British Journal of Social Work*, 35, 1093–106.

Wright, P, Turner, C, Clay, D and Mills, H (2006) Participation of children and young people in developing social care. *Practice Guide 06*. London: Social Care Institute for Excellence.

Yukl, G (1989) Managerial leadership: a review of theory and research. *Journal of Management,* 16, 254–89.

Index

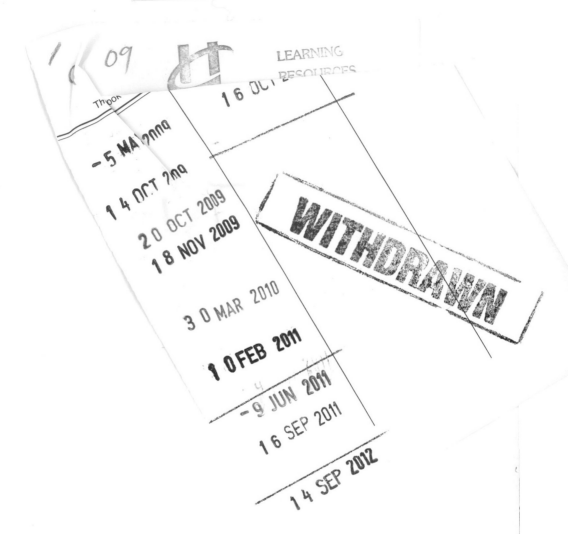

LEARNING RESOURCES

-5 MAR 2009

1 4 OCT 2009

2 0 OCT 2009

1 8 NOV 2009

3 0 MAR 2010

1 0 FEB 2011

-9 JUN 2011

1 6 SEP 2011

1 4 SEP 2012

1 6 OCT

WITHDRAWN

For enquiries or renewal at
Quarles LRC
Tel: 01708 455011 – Extension 4009